Palliative Skills for Frontline Clinicians

Kate Aberger • David Wang

Editors

Palliative Skills for Frontline Clinicians

Case Vignettes in Everyday Hospital Medicine

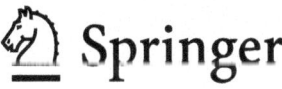

Editors
Kate Aberger
Director of Palliative and Geriatric Medicine
St. Joseph's Health
Paterson, NJ
USA

David Wang
Director of Palliative Medicine
Scripps Health
San Diego, CA
USA

Attending Physician, Emergency
Department Robert Wood Johnson
University Hospital
Somerset, NJ
USA

ISBN 978-3-030-44413-6   ISBN 978-3-030-44414-3   (eBook)
https://doi.org/10.1007/978-3-030-44414-3

This Springer imprint is published by the registered company Springer Nature Switzerland AG
The registered company address is: Gewerbestrasse 11, 6330 Cham, Switzerland

To our patients and their families: thank you for your vulnerability and for allowing us to learn how to best care for you.

Foreword

Our health-care system has an urgent need for clinicians who are skilled in integrating palliative care practices into their everyday care for patients with serious illness. The specialty of Hospice and Palliative Medicine will remain too small to assure that all patients with serious illness have access to these palliative approaches. All clinicians who care for seriously ill patients will benefit from learning fundamental, patient-centered palliative care competencies relevant to their own practice settings. This terrific new resource, *Palliative Skills for Frontline Clinicians: Case Vignettes in Everyday Hospital Medicine*, demonstrates how this can be done in a practical and realistic way.

The authors, all experts in disciplines that range from Emergency Medicine to Primary Care and Internal Medicine subspecialties to Obstetrics and Gynecology and Pediatrics and Surgery, describe their common clinical cases. Each case is followed by two different pathways – the conventional approach to treating the disease, in which considerations of diagnosis, treatment options, risks, and benefits and potential impact on morbidity and mortality determine therapeutic decisions, and the palliative approach, in which these considerations are balanced with an equal focus on the patient's goals and values, acceptable and unacceptable tradeoffs, quality-of-life considerations, and family needs. Examples of communication strategies that would be useful for each vignette are included, as well as palliative symptom management techniques that could benefit the patient. Clinicians come away with both new ways of thinking about integrating this approach and basic competencies to help them achieve this goal.

This book is based on a simple yet profound observation: the best treatment plans integrate medical considerations (diagnosis treatment options, risks and benefits, impact on outcomes) with an understanding of what matters to the patient (through elicitation of values and goals, understanding of tradeoffs the patient is and is not willing to make, appreciation of the patient's perspective on acceptable quality of life, and awareness of family needs). Our current health-care system gives primacy to the medical goals while subordinating the personal values and goals of patients. Each of these approaches alone is insufficient to assure that the patient will receive high-quality care.

This book shows how to actualize this aspiration of integration in a wide variety of clinical scenarios, within the constraints of the real-world practice of medicine. This approach will benefit patients and their families and, just as importantly, the clinicians who learn it. Clinicians will develop a broader repertoire of competencies that allow them to practice the kind of medicine they envisioned when they went into the field of medicine. This work is a terrific contribution to the field.

Susan Block
Dana-Farber Cancer Institute, Brigham and Women's Hospital
Boston, MA, USA

Preface

Over the course of clinical training, we develop agendas in treatment and disposition which come to outweigh listening to our patients. The practice of modern medicine perpetuates algorithmic treatments with relentless, checklist efficiency. When care doesn't fit neatly into these boxes, both clinicians and patients (and their families) feel frustrated. What open dialogue might have addressed is now often displaced by busyness and external health system forces. How can clinicians meet patients with serious illness where they are while also balancing the realities of our jobs?

We present this work as one means to realign ourselves with our patients. This book is written *by you* and *for you*. These authors all care for patients in the specialties and settings they write about and additionally have palliative care training or certification. Palliative skills are anchored in patient-centered care and widely applicable across medicine beyond its own subspecialty. Our authors present challenging case vignettes (adapted from real patients) that are frequently encountered in hospital settings. Using narrative language, they describe both how care usually progresses and introduce an alternative, palliative-embedded approach to patients and their families. Through these vignettes, you will acquire actionable communication and symptom management strategies to turn your most trying cases into fulfilling ones.

Read this book as a collection of short stories. This is not a textbook; many palliative aspects are better shown than told. You will find phraseology, frameworks, and scripting to walk you through new communication styles. Callout boxes and take-away points highlight each case's key message. There is at times intentional redundancy, because these principles apply irrespective of patient disease or clinical specialty.

We now learn a more comprehensive way of thinking and communicating. We investigate everything about the disease while simultaneously, with just as much intention, we deeply explore the lives of our patients and families. We then present recommendations based on the synthesis of these two dimensions: the disease's process, prognosis, and morbidity *and* the patient's values, fears, and hopes. This realigns us with our patients and families and truly defines patient-centered care: the right care at the right time in the right place. Let us go and reclaim the sacred physician-patient relationship.

Paterson, NJ, USA   Kate Aberger
San Diego, CA, USA   David Wang

Acknowledgments

Dr. Kate Aberger acknowledges her mother, Julianna Aberger, for her support and copyediting of this work, as well as her family – Richard, Maye, Rory, Melissa, and assorted cats, dogs, and fish – for keeping this life worthwhile.

Dr. David Wang is grateful to his wife, Judy, for her steadfast encouragement, and their son, Desmond, a gift and miracle.

We honor our mentors in both emergency medicine and palliative medicine for continuously challenging us to enrich our practice of the art of medicine.

Contents

Contributors

Kate Aberger, MD Division of Palliative Medicine and Geriatrics, St. Joseph's University Medical Center, Paterson, NJ, USA

Emergency Department, Robert Wood Johnson University Hospital Somerset, Somerville, NJ, USA

Josephine Amory, MD Maternal Fetal Medicine, Palliative Medicine, University of Washington, Seattle, WA, USA

Ana Berlin, MD, MPH Surgery (Acute Care Surgery) and Medicine (Adult Palliative Medicine), Columbia University Irving Medical Center, New York, NY, USA

Jessica Besbris, MD Department of Neurology, Department of Supportive Care Medicine, Cedars-Sinai Medical Center, Los Angeles, CA, USA

Jason K. Bowman, MD Department of Emergency Medicine, Massachusetts General Hospital, Boston, MA, USA

Department of Emergency Medicine, Harvard Medical School, Boston, MA, USA

Department of Emergency Medicine, Brigham and Women's Hospital, Boston, MA, USA

William Burns, MD BerbeeWalsh Department of Emergency Medicine, Division of Hematology, Medical Oncology, and Palliative Care, University of Wisconsin School of Medicine & Public Health, Madison, WI, USA

T. Johelen Carleton, MD Medical Director Palliative Care, Tucson Medical Center, Tucson, AZ, USA

Ann Marie Case, MD Pediatrics, Palliative Medicine, Dell Children's Medical Center of Central Texas, Austin, TX, USA

Rachel Danczyk, MD University of New Mexico Department of Surgery, Albuquerque VA Medical Center, Albuquerque, NM, USA

Indra D. Daniels, MD Nephrology and Hospice & Palliative Medicine, Attending Physician, Palliative Care Service Mount Sinai South Nassau, Oceanside, NY, USA

Clinical Assistant Professor of Medicine, Icahn School of Medicine at Mount Sinai, Oceanside, NY, USA

Andrew Epstein, MD Supportive Care Service, Memorial Sloan Kettering Cancer Center, New York, NY, USA

Gastrointestinal Oncology Service, Memorial Sloan Kettering Cancer Center, New York, NY, USA

Department of Medicine, Weill Cornell Medical College, New York, NY, USA

Brandon Francis, MD, MPH Department of Neurology and Ophthalmology, Stroke and Neurocritical Care Services, Michigan State University, East Lansing, MI, USA

Jennifer Y. Fung, MD Department of Medicine, Mount Sinai Morningside, New York, NY, USA

Alan Garber, MD Department of Medicine, Mary Imogene Bassett Hospital, Cooperstown, NY, USA

Lauren Goodman, MD Department of Internal Medicine, Division of Pulmonary, Critical Care and Sleep, The Ohio State University Wexner Medical Center, Columbus, OH, USA

Calista M. Harbaugh, MD, MS Department of Surgery, University of Michigan, Ann Arbor, MI, USA

Bridget Highet, MD Halifax Health Department of Emergency Medicine, Halifax Health Hospice, Daytona Beach, FL, USA

Daniel B. Hinshaw, MD Palliative Care Program, University of Michigan Geriatrics Center, Ann Arbor, MI, USA

Melissa Red Hoffman, MD, ND Department of Surgery, Mission Hospital, Asheville, NC, USA

Marynell Jelinek, MD, FACEP Department of Emergency Medicine, USC Keck School of Medicine, LAC+USC Medical Center, Los Angeles, CA, USA

Jaime Jump, DO Department of Pediatrics-Sections of Critical Care and Palliative Care, Texas Children's Hospital, Houston, TX, USA

Erika Ketteler, MD Raymond G. Murphy VAMC, Albuquerque, NM, USA

Krishelle Marc-Aurele, MD Neonatology, Palliative Medicine, University of California, San Diego, CA, USA

Emily Jean Martin, MD Palliative Care Program, Department of Medicine, UCLA David Geffen School of Medicine, Los Angeles, CA, USA

Kevin McGehrin, MD Department of Neurosciences, University of California – San Diego, San Diego, CA, USA

Pringl Miller, MD, FACS Departments of Medicine and Surgery, Rush University Medical Center, Chicago, IL, USA

Andrea K. Nagengast, MD Department of Surgery, Oregon Health and Science University, Portland, OR, USA

Carter Neugarten, MD Palliative Medicine and Emergency Medicine, Rush University, Chicago, IL, USA

Kei Ouchi, MD, MPH Department of Emergency Medicine, Harvard Medical School, Boston, MA, USA

Department of Emergency Medicine, Brigham and Women's Hospital, Boston, MA, USA

Rushil Patel, MD Supportive Care Service, Memorial Sloan Kettering Cancer Center, New York, NY, USA

Alison Petok, MPH, MSW Private Practice, Jamaica Plain, MA, USA

Joel Phillips, DO Hauenstein Neurosciences, Mercy Health Saint Mary's Hospital, Michigan State University, Grand Rapids, MI, USA

Jay A. Requarth, MD Wake Forest School of Medicine, Winston Salem, NC, USA

Nathan M. Riley, MD Obstetrics and Gynecology, Palliative Medicine, Norton Healthcare, Louisville, KY, USA

Tamara Rubenzik, MD Departments of Nephrology and Palliative Care, University of California San Diego, San Diego, CA, USA

Christopher P. Scally, MD, MS Department of Surgical Oncology, University of Texas M.D. Anderson Cancer Center, Houston, TX, USA

Monique Schaulis, MD, MPH The Permanente Medical Group, San Francisco, CA, USA

Neha Shah, MD, FIDSA Piedmont Healthcare, Georgia, GA, USA

Cara Siegel, MD UCLA Department of Neurology, Los Angeles, CA, USA

Pasithorn A. Suwanabol, MD, MS Department of Surgery, University of Michigan, Ann Arbor, MI, USA

Audrey Tan, DO Ronald O. Perelman Department of Emergency Medicine, Department of Internal Medicine, New York University School of Medicine, New York, NY, USA

Christine Toevs, MD Terre Haute Regional Hospital, Terre Haute, IN, USA

Nitin Ubhayakar, MD Emergency Medicine Physician, White Memorial Hospital, Los Angeles, CA, USA

Palliative Care Physician, Huntington Memorial Hospital, Pasadena, CA, USA

Christina L. Vaughan, MD, MHS Department of Neurology, Section of Neuro-Palliative Care, University of Colorado, Anschutz Medical Campus, Aurora, CO, USA

Department of Medicine, Palliative Care Inpatient Consult Service, University of Colorado Hospital, Aurora, CO, USA

Justin Voorhees, MD, MSc Hospice of Lenawee, Advian, MI, USA

David Wang, MD Palliative Medicine, Scripps Health, San Diego, CA, USA

Evan Wong, MDiv, BCC Department of Palliative Care, Kaiser Permanente, Fremont, CA, USA

Brooke Worster, MD, FACP Department of Medical Oncology, Thomas Jefferson University Hospital/Sidney Kimmel Cancer Center, Philadelphia, PA, USA

David Zonies, MD, MPH Department of Surgery, Oregon Health and Science University, Portland, OR, USA

Abbreviations

ACEP	American College of Emergency Physicians
ACS	American College of Surgeons
ADL	Activity of daily living
AKI	Acute kidney injury
ANH	Artificial nutrition and hydration
ARDS	Acute respiratory distress syndrome
AV	Arteriovenous
BC/WC	Best case/worst case
BiPAP	Bilevel positive airway pressure
BP	Blood pressure
CKD	Chronic kidney disease
COPD	Chronic obstructive pulmonary disease
CPR	Cardiopulmonary resuscitation
CRRT	Continuous renal replacement therapy
CSF	Cerebrospinal fluid
CT	CAT scan
CTA	CAT Scan Angiography
CVVH	Continuous veno-venous hemofiltration
DNI	Do not intubate
DNR	Do not resuscitate
DuoNebs	Ipratropium bromide and albuterol sulfate
DVT	Deep vein thrombosis
ECOG	Eastern Cooperative Oncology Group
ED	Emergency department
EF	Ejection fraction
EGD	Esophagogastroduodenoscopy
EMR	Electronic medical record
ESAS	Edmonton Symptom Assessment Scale
ESAS-R	Edmonton Symptom Assessment Scale-Revised
ESRD	End-stage renal disease
FiO2	Fraction of inspired oxygen

GCS	Glasgow Coma Scale
HCP	Health-care proxy
HCPOA	Health-care power of attorney
HFNC	High-flow nasal canula
HR	Heart rate
Hr	Hour
ICU	Intensive care unit
IPU	Inpatient unit
IV	Intravenous
IVF	Intravenous fluids
L	Liter
LTACH	Long-term acute care hospital
MAT	Medication-assisted treatment
MFM	Maternal-fetal medicine
Mg	Milligram
mmol	Millimole
MOLST	Medical Orders for Life-Sustaining Treatment
MRI	Magnetic resonance imaging
MRSA	Methicillin-resistant *Staphylococcus aureus*
MS Contin	Morphine sulfate
NG	Nasogastric
NICU	Neonatal intensive care unit
NMDA	N-methyl-D-aspartate
NMDAR	N-methyl-D-aspartate receptor
NPO	Nil per os
NPPV	Noninvasive positive pressure ventilation
NSAIDs	Nonsteroidal anti-inflammatory
NSQIP	National Surgical Quality Improvement Program
O2	Oxygen
OME	Oral morphine equivalents
OR	Operating room
OUD	Opiate use disorder
PACU	Post-anesthesia care unit
PD	Parkinson's disease
PEEP	Peak end-expiratory pressure
PEG	Percutaneous endoscopic gastrostomy
PET	Positron emission tomography
PICC	Peripherally inserted central catheter
PICU	Pediatric intensive care unit
POD	Postoperative day
POLST	Physician Order for Life-Sustaining Treatment
PRN	Pro re nata
RASS	Richmond Agitation-Sedation Score
ROSC	Return of spontaneous circulation
RPA	Renal Physicians Association

RR	Respiratory rate
Sat	Saturation
SDM	Shared decision-making
SpO2	Peripheral capillary oxygen saturation
SUD	Substance use disorder
T	Temperature
T18	Trisomy 18
TAVR	Transcatheter aortic valve replacement
TLT	Time-limited trial
TPA	Tissue plasminogen activator
TPN	Total parenteral nutrition
Trach	Tracheostomy
umol	Micromole
VA	Veterans Affairs
WBC	White blood cells
XRT	Radiation therapy

Part I
Emergency Medicine

Chapter 1
High-Yield Approach to the ED Goals of Care Conversation

Bridget Highet

Case Introduction

Emergency Medical Services (EMS) transports a frail 78-year-old male to the emergency department. Wearing BiPAP (bilevel positive airway pressure), he is gasping and using accessory muscles. He responds poorly. The paramedic states: "The nursing home found him with shortness of breath this morning. When we arrived his baseline SpO_2 was 70% on 6 liters nasal cannula. We have given him three DuoNebs, 125 mg of methylprednisolone, and started him on BiPAP. We have only been able to get him to 76%. They say he has lung disease; he has no DNR or POLST. His daughter is on the way."

The patient is dying of respiratory failure. You perform rapid sequence intubation. Following intubation, his oxygen saturation continues to fluctuate between 80% and 84% despite 100% FiO_2 and positive end expiratory pressure (PEEP) of 15.

The patient's medical record reveals that 4 years ago, a pulmonologist diagnosed idiopathic pulmonary fibrosis. Over the past year, his lung function has declined, with his supplemental oxygen needs increasing from two liters to six within the past 6 months. One year ago, he was moved into a skilled nursing facility because he was unable to care for himself.

Standard Approach

Labs are obtained, a chest X-ray is ordered, and the patient is optimized on mechanical ventilation. The family is called and provided a medical update on the patient's critical condition. The patient is admitted to the intensive care unit for continued management.

B. Highet (✉)
Halifax Health Department of Emergency Medicine, Halifax Health Hospice,
Daytona Beach, FL, USA

© Springer Nature Switzerland AG 2020
K. Aberger, D. Wang (eds.), *Palliative Skills for Frontline Clinicians*,
https://doi.org/10.1007/978-3-030-44414-3_1

Palliative Approach

This patient is seriously ill; when he came in, he looked like he was dying. His pulmonary fibrosis is an irreversible condition, and based on his chart, he has had a significant functional decline in the past year. Even if he survives this hospital stay, his best-case scenario would be to return to the nursing home, likely with more limited function than he has now.

The patient's daughter is listed as his primary contact. You call and ask what she knows so far. She tells you she knows he is in the hospital, and that he is very sick. She is on her way to the ED. You use simple language, explaining to her that he is on "life support" and you are worried that he is "dying." You expect and allow space for an emotional response.

Box 1.1 There Is no Substitute for "Dying"

The first step in navigating a palliative approach at the end of life is choosing the right words. When we describe someone as having severe hypoxic respiratory failure, might we also say that the patient is dying of lung disease? The operative word is dying, and not "expiring," "passing," "leaving," or "not surviving." No decision can be made if ambiguity and misunderstanding remain.

Several studies have demonstrated that physicians often fall back on euphemisms or indirect language when discussing death [1, 2]. Recognizing impending death and communicating this to family members is not a part of our culture or training, but it is imperative to high-quality end-of-life discussions in the acute setting.

You establish that the patient's daughter is his health-care surrogate. She informs you that the patient is widowed, and she is his only child.

Box 1.2 Who Is the Best Surrogate?

When a patient lacks capacity to speak for themselves, it is important to identify the most appropriate surrogate prior to engaging in goals of care conversations. When no power of attorney has been legally appointed, decisional hierarchy law varies across states, ranging from rigid surrogacy ladders (e.g., first spouse, then in order children, parents, siblings, etc.) to undefined priority order for persons [3]. Advance care planning documents that limit life-sustaining treatments (e.g., POLST, MOLST, advance directives) must be upheld in the emergency department as legal documents and can serve as effective conversation starters. The most recently notarized/signed document is most valid.

You ask, "Can you tell me about your father? What kind of person is he?".

You hear the timbre in her voice change. She responds: "What can I say? He is an amazing person. My mom died when I was young, and he raised me on his own. He has always been someone people can count on. He worked as an engineer for 40 years for the same company. He loves doing projects, and staying busy. He hates being sick. He hates the nursing home."

You thank her for painting this vivid picture of him, and explore further saying: "This must be hard. What do you think he would say if he could see himself on life support?"

She responds: "We have talked about it. He never wanted to be kept alive on machines. He said when it was his time, 'let me go'. My mother died of cancer. She had a horrible death. She was on machines – she died in the hospital. My father regretted it so much. He would never want a death like that."

Box 1.3 The Conversation Is About More Than Medicine

This demonstrates two valuable communication techniques in eliciting the goals and values of a patient. The first is inquiring "What kind of person is your father?" or "Tell me about your father." Families will often open up and describe the values of their loved one, allowing you to make a recommendation that is most in line with the patient's wishes. The second technique is to bring the patient to the bedside. "If your father could speak to us right now, what would he say?" Exploring this allows the family, in their role as surrogate, to make the decisions most aligned with the patient's wishes and values [4, 5].

You now believe that she is prepared to make a decision: "I know this all must be very difficult to hear. Is it ok if I talk with you about our options from here and make a recommendation?"

"Yes, that would be ok."

"It sounds like your father valued his independence and didn't like being sick. He saw your mother struggle on life support, and it's not something he would want at the end of his life. While we could continue life support and admit your father to the ICU, I worry this isn't in line with his wishes. My recommendation is that we discontinue his life support and allow him to die naturally and comfortably."

Box 1.4 You Should First Make a Recommendation Before Asking for a Decision

Based on the values elicited earlier in the conversation, you make a recommendation that takes into account the patient's wishes [6]. Clinicians know there are many treatment options for this patient — more time on the ventilator, central line and vasopressors, CPR or DNR, antibiotics — but from the information we have elicited from this family member, it is clear that one of these options is the most aligned with the patient's wishes. While we often are comfortable making recommendations regarding medicines or treatments, we struggle with assertiveness at the end of life.

Physicians should not shy away from recommendations. Families are relying on us to process the variables and give them our opinion. Our medical knowledge and experience is essential to patients and families when they are processing the complexities of these difficult choices. By synthesizing what we know about a patient with our medical expertise, we can guide families in the difficult choices they are faced with at the end of life.

As the gravity of the moment starts to sink in, his daughter asks: "But are you sure he is dying? How can you be sure? What if this isn't pulmonary fibrosis at all? I had an aunt who had cancer and the hospital missed it for years. She died and they could have saved her if they had caught it earlier. I was reading about a new drug for pulmonary fibrosis. Maybe we could try that?"

You say, "This must be really hard to hear."

Box 1.5 Often Saying Less Is More, and Allow Room for Silence
Patients and families often communicate emotions to us through their questions. Physicians often miss opportunities to validate and respond to emotion [7]. A common pitfall would be to respond to this patient's question with medical talk, explaining to her why this won't work or explaining how that isn't an option. Medical talk will bury your empathy, and it often isn't what the family is searching for. Using an empathetic statement like "This must be really hard to hear" allows you to acknowledge that emotion and provide space for the family to process what is going on.

You allow 10 seconds to pass in silence as she emotionally digests the situation. Although this may feel like an eternity, patients and surrogates significantly benefit from having this space. "Yes, this is really hard. I can't believe this is where we are. But, you are right. He always said he would never want to be on life support."

"This is really difficult, and we will support you in this. Let's talk more about the next steps when you arrive."

You inform the charge nurse of the situation, and ask her to have the chaplain called, and to involve the social worker to contact hospice.

Box 1.6 Preparing for a Palliative Disposition
It is very difficult to predict the trajectories of patients following withdrawal of mechanical ventilation. While many patients will only survive minutes to hours, some may survive several days [8]. It is important to prepare for this

and to counsel the family regarding this uncertainty. Involving hospice services in a terminal extubation may allow a discharge plan for the patient if the patient survives and can also engage important resources for families like bereavement support following the patient's death.

It is also important for physicians to familiarize themselves with the statutes in the region in which they are practicing, and their own hospital policies regarding withdrawal of life-sustaining measures. Some states have specific documentation requirements and mandate one or two physicians to certify in writing that the patient is in an end-stage or terminal condition. Most hospitals have these forms easily available, and the palliative care physician or intensivist can assist in certifying a patient's condition if the statute requires an additional physician's exam.

The charge nurse moves the patient to a quieter corner of the emergency department. She places a placard on the door to alert staff that a compassionate extubation may be taking place so as to minimize room traffic.

The daughter arrives. You introduce her to the patient's nurse, chaplain, social worker, and respiratory therapist. She feels comfortable with the plan to discontinue the ventilator. You walk her through the process, including premedication to help mitigate any breathlessness or anxiety. You warn her that he may appear to gurgle (pooling secretions) after the tube is out, and that while hard to see, it is not directly distressing to him. You reassure her that you will aggressively treat any discomfort. You also inform her that you are placing a "Do Not Resuscitate" order in the chart so that her father may die naturally.

You turn off the monitors in the room. You note to yourself that the patient received succinylcholine 2 hours prior but has not received any other paralytic agents. You administer 0.4 mg glycopyrrolate IV to prevent secretions following extubation. You then administer a bolus of 2 mg of morphine IV and 2 mg of midazolam IV, and you turn off the patient's Propofol. You step out of the room and return to reassess the patient 10 minutes later. He appears comfortable with no evidence of anxiety or dyspnea. You step down the patient's PEEP from 15 to 5 and decrease his FiO_2 to 50%. You return ten minutes later and find the patient grimacing. You administer an additional 4 mg of IV morphine. Upon reassessment, the patient appears comfortable. You place the patient on pressure support. The patient continues to appear comfortable on reassessment.

The endotracheal tube is now removed. The patient appears peaceful, with no grimacing or anxiety. His daughter chooses to stay by his side during the extubation.

The nurse comes and gets you 30 minutes later. The patient has a furrowed brow, is breathing quickly, and looks uncomfortable. You assess that he appears anxious and administer an additional bolus of 2 mg of midazolam IV. On reassessment, 15 minutes later the patient is resting comfortably and his breathing and facial expression have eased (Table 1.1).

The patient continues to breathe comfortably. He is somnolent but demonstrates no signs of distress. Given the likelihood of requiring escalating parenteral

Table 1.1 Compassionate extubation should proceed systematically

Step	Consideration
1. Ensure no recent paralytics given.	They may mask distress peri-extubation.
2. Establish a quiet setting (e.g., discontinue monitoring, place sign on room, provide space for family).	
3. Administer anticholinergic (glycopyrrolate, atropine, etc.) well in advance of extubation.	They do not dry up existing secretions, but may help prevent formation of new secretions. The evidence is inconclusive. However, there are few adverse effects and may mitigate family distress from hearing the "death rattle" [9].
4. Premedicate with bolus of opioid for dyspnea and benzodiazepine for anxiety.	Many physicians are concerned that opiates or benzodiazepines at the end of life may hasten death. However, multiple studies have demonstrated that the use of these medicines in symptomatic treatment at the end of life has not been shown to impact survival [10].
5. Consider weaning ventilator support settings stepwise and with reassessment for symptoms and additional medication as necessary.	Low tidal volumes on high support portend high likelihood of air hunger and medication requirement. Gradual weaning reduces magnitude of distress [11]. Immediate extubation without weaning has been correlated with airway obstruction and higher pain scores [12].
6. Have additional medication doses readily available peri-extubation.	Having your nurse leave the bedside to retrieve more doses may be very distressing to family already witnessing their loved one experience air hunger.
7. Extubate. Continue to administer opioids and benzodiazepines for symptoms.	Dosing can be repeated every 10 minutes and doubled to achieve dyspnea or pain control.

medication, you admit him to General Inpatient Hospice. You do this only after further discussion with his daughter who is thankful for your support, as she cannot care for him at home. Several days later, the patient dies.

Take-Away Points
1. Recognize dying patients in the emergency department, and avoid euphemisms in discussing death with families.
2. Elicit a patient's wishes and values, and then issue clear recommendations based on these.
3. Saying less is more, allow room for silence.
4. Approach compassionate extubation as a systematic procedure, integrating family and whole-team preparation.

References

1. Rodriguez KL, et al. Pushing up daisies: implicit and explicit language in oncologist-patient communication about death. Support Care Cancer. 2007;15(2):153–61.
2. Collins A, McLachlan SA, Philip J. Communication about palliative care: a phenomenological study exploring patient views and responses to its discussion. Palliat Med. 2018;32(1):133–42.
3. DeMartino ES, et al. Who decides when a patient can't? Statutes on alternate decision makers. N Engl J Med. 2017;376(15):1478–82.
4. Cook D, Rocker G. Dying with dignity in the intensive care unit. N Engl J Med. 2014;370(26):2506–14.
5. Berlin A. Goals of care and end of life in the ICU. Surg Clin North Am. 2017;97(6):1275–90.
6. Childers JW, et al. REMAP: a framework for goals of care conversations. J Oncol Pract. 2017;13(10):e844–50.
7. Curtis JR, et al. Missed opportunities during family conferences about end-of-life care in the intensive care unit. Am J Respir Crit Care Med. 2005;171(8):844–9.
8. Cooke CR, et al. Predictors of time to death after terminal withdrawal of mechanical ventilation in the ICU. Chest. 2010;138(2):289–97.
9. Lokker ME, et al. Prevalence, impact, and treatment of death rattle: a systematic review. J Pain Symptom Manag. 2014;47(1):105–22.
10. Sykes N, Thorns A. The use of opioids and sedatives at the end of life. Lancet Oncol. 2003;4(5):312–8.
11. Wang D, Creel-Bulos C. A systematic approach to comfort care transitions in the emergency department. J Emerg Med. 2019;56(3):267–74. https://doi.org/10.1016/j.jemermed.2018.10.027.
12. Robert R, et al. Terminal weaning or immediate extubation for withdrawing mechanical ventilation in critically ill patients (the ARREVE observational study). Intensive Care Med. 2017;43(12):1793–807.

Chapter 2
A Palliative Approach to End-Stage COPD

Carter Neugarten and William Burns

Case Introduction

Rose is a 75-year-old woman who presents to the ED with the chief complaint of shortness of breath. A brief review of her medical record reveals that she has a history of severe chronic obstructive pulmonary disease (COPD) requiring two liters of supplemental oxygen at home, as well as a lengthy history of anxiety. She has had seven hospitalizations for COPD exacerbations in the past four months and was most recently discharged two weeks ago. During this last admission, she was intubated for several days after failing a trial of noninvasive positive pressure ventilation. Her triage note today indicates that she has been increasingly short of breath over the past few days.

Rose is able to provide a clear history of similar symptoms of her past COPD exacerbations, and you note that she pauses midway through sentences to catch her breath. She tells you that she typically waits until symptoms worsen to present to the ED, but today she does not want a breathing tube, as happened last time. At home, she had been taking all her medications as prescribed and was using her nebulizers every four hours. However, she was unable to control her dyspnea. She denies any changes to her sputum, fever, chest pain, orthopnea, or leg swelling. On exam, she is tachypneic and has mildly increased work of breathing. She also has diffusely poor air entry and wheezing. Her triage electrocardiogram is at its baseline.

C. Neugarten (✉)
Palliative Medicine and Emergency Medicine, Rush University, Chicago, IL, USA

W. Burns
BerbeeWalsh Department of Emergency Medicine, Division of Hematology, Medical Oncology, and Palliative Care, University of Wisconsin School of Medicine & Public Health, Madison, WI, USA

© Springer Nature Switzerland AG 2020
K. Aberger, D. Wang (eds.), *Palliative Skills for Frontline Clinicians*,
https://doi.org/10.1007/978-3-030-44414-3_2

Usual Approach

At this point, Rose does not appear to be critically ill but is failing outpatient management. The standard ED approach would be to pursue screening labs and chest radiograph, administer steroids and continuous nebulizers, perhaps start BiPAP, and admit her for further care.

You might also ask briefly about a patient's code status, something such as: "If your heart stops, do you want us to put a tube down your throat, push on your chest, and use electricity to try to restart it?"

Palliative Approach

There is a cohort of chronically ill patients such as Rose whose diagnoses, treatment plans, and dispositions are immediately apparent to the experienced ED clinician. Such clinically straightforward cases are often quickly and efficiently treated by an ED provider. However, these are also patients in whom even short interventions, or exploration of a patient's goals, may prevent unwanted care and save time for the patient and providers who care for them in the future.

Emergency providers sometimes feel that it is not their responsibility to explore goals of care with patients in the ED, and that they do not have the time to do so. However, all health-care providers share this responsibility, and sometimes patients do not have adequate outpatient care for these issues to be addressed before they arrive in the hospital. Furthermore, decisions we make in the ED, including intubation and ICU admission, put these patients on a trajectory of care that may not be in line with their preferences.

In this case, Rose made clear that she presented earlier in her COPD exacerbation to avoid intubation. Her ED provider is thus presented with a choice. While providers are often taught to use open-ended questions when initially interviewing patients about their symptoms, time constraints in the ED often create pressure to revert to closed-ended questions to obtain the necessary clinical information. When interviewing patients about their wishes and goals of care, however, open-ended questions are often more effective. Imagine asking this patient the following question:

Rose, I noticed that you said you came in early because last night you were worried about needing a breathing tube again. Will you tell me more about that?

Box 2.1 "Tell Me More"
Simply saying "Tell me more," or a variation of this phrase, is a powerful tool to elicit detail about a patient's emotions.

Table 2.1 Two approaches to ED goals of care conversations

Usual approach	Palliative approach
Provider: *If your heart stops, do you want us to put a tube in your mouth, push on your chest, and use electricity to try to restart it?* Patient: *Yes, of course I want you to do everything.*	Provider: *What scares you about your illness?* Patient: *I don't want to suffer, and I don't want to end up on all those machines with tubes coming out of me from everywhere.* Provider: *Tell me more about what you mean by that.*
Provider: *Are you okay with being in the ICU and having medicines to artificially keep up your blood pressure through a large IV in your neck?* Patient: *What other choice do I have? You do whatever you have to.*	Provider: *Have you thought about what you would want the end of your life to look like?* Patient: *Well, I guess I would want to be at home, with my family and loved ones.*

In response, Rose relates that she cannot remember all the time she was on the ventilator, but she does remember some parts vividly. In specific, she recalls being awake when they took it out and how uncomfortable and horrifying that experience was. She relates that she has been having nightmares about not being able to breathe and wonders if she really needed to be awake when it was removed. Finally, she states she is hoping she came in early enough to avoid the trauma of intubation.

You can identify a number of important issues by listening closely to Rose's response. Imagine how much of her response would have been missed if the conversation had been cut short after Rose described how uncomfortable the extubation was (Table 2.1).

When responding to emotion, responses from a provider might include phrases such as "I understand," "that won't happen again," or "it will be okay." There is no single best way to respond when someone discloses traumatic experiences, as patients will often have unique experiences and emotions. In reality, while it is important to express empathy, we cannot truly understand another person's personal experience, and there is little about the future that we can guarantee. However, we can always validate their experience, and one response that can often be effective is "I can't imagine how horrible that must have been."

Sometimes empathic statements such as these allow a conversation to continue immediately, while at other times they are followed by a pause.

Box 2.2 The Power of Silence
There is profound power in silence, and a provider's patience is often rewarded. It may feel like a great deal of time has passed, but the time is usually much shorter. Many things may be happening during the silence. The patient may be deciding whether to trust you with something they have not let themselves say out loud. They may be coming to a realization they had not expected or considered before. Or, they may be composing themselves to make a serious decision. At the same time, by providing them space, you are building rapport and giving them time to focus on matters of consequence to them.

When you use empathic statements and provide Rose with silence to think and respond, she thanks you and notes that not all doctors really listen. She explains that she has been thinking about dying and worries that her life is not going to get better. She does not want to spend the rest of her life in the hospital, but fears the feeling of suffocation. Finally, she appreciates your time, but she does not want to make any decisions without her daughter present, who is her medical power of attorney.

In this situation, Rose provided a window into her personal experience and details her fears and goals, as well as her decision-making process. A provider might be tempted to push this patient to engage in a discussion about code status at that moment, but there is a risk that this discussion may be premature and may damage rapport with the patient. The absence of effecting, or even introducing, code status does not reduce the significant value of this conversation. Instead, the critical next steps are to encourage the patient to discuss these issues with her daughter if she has not already done so, document the conversation in the patient's chart, and alert the accepting inpatient provider that the patient is considering placing limitations on her care. If the patient subsequently loses her ability to make decisions, details such as these can provide significant background and support to a patient's family, critical care teams, and palliative care providers.

Family members often err on the side of "doing more" for their loved ones if these conversations have not taken place before a patient loses capacity, or if pertinent information has not been discussed. Medical powers of attorney can experience significant emotional burden and guilt when placing limitations on care they had not heard the patient express. Having knowledge of a patient's prior wishes allows family members to make better informed decisions without experiencing unnecessary guilt.

Case Continued

Rose was admitted to the floor and she improved clinically. She avoided intubation and returned home to spend quality time with her family. Two months later, you arrive at your shift and notice that your colleague is taking care of Rose. This time, she arrived in respiratory distress and was found to have a severe COPD exacerbation. She was given continuous nebs, steroids, and placed on BiPAP. Unfortunately, she is not improving and is now altered, secondary to hypercapnia.

Usual Approach

Your colleague makes the decision to intubate her. Later, her daughter arrives and reports that Rose would not have wanted this, but she feels guilty about extubating her, so her mother is transferred to the ICU. She becomes progressively hypercarbic and difficult to ventilate. Several days later, she dies on the ventilator in the ICU.

Palliative Approach

Your colleague was able to identify the appropriate medical power of attorney to call, because you included her daughter's name and phone number in your documentation. Her daughter reports that she has spoken multiple times to Rose about what she would, and would not, want at the end of her life. Rose's daughter elects comfort-focused care based on her current clinical condition. Rose is admitted to a medical floor, and her dyspnea is controlled with low-dose morphine. She is able to return home the next day with the support of hospice, and later dies, surrounded by her family. They are grateful for the care provided, and that she was able to be at home and not have her dying process artificially prolonged.

Box 2.3 Correct Dosage of Opioids for Dyspnea

A common palliative treatment of dyspnea is to use opioids. The starting dose for treatment of dyspnea is often lower than what is used for treating pain. For example, a starting dose of 2.5 mg oral morphine solution can be given every 4 hours as needed for dyspnea (or approximately 1 mg IV morphine every hour). Since morphine should be avoided in patients with renal dysfunction, 1 mg of oral hydromorphone (or 0.25 mg IV) could also be considered.

Take-Away Points

1. Goals of care conversations do not need to contain a discussion about code status. Rather, they should focus on what is important to the patient in view of what is happening clinically at that time. Eliciting patients' priorities and values can help enlighten a provider's recommendations on issues such as code status. These do not need to be long conversations, and even spending a few minutes initiating these conversations in the ED can pay large dividends in the future.
2. Be open to listening to the patient's own understanding, fears, goals, and experiences.
3. There is profound power in silence. Pauses can be one of the most effective tools when participating in difficult conversations. Do not interrupt.
4. Document patients' preferences for limitations on their care. This information substantiates future decision-making for both families and providers.

Chapter 3
This POLST Makes No Sense

Jason K. Bowman and Kei Ouchi

Case Introduction

An 87-year-old male with dementia (oriented to name only) is brought in by ambulance from a memory care facility after several days of fever, productive cough, bilateral leg swelling, and worsening hypoxia. Paramedics hand you a POLST (Physician Orders for Life-Sustaining Treatment) form that was signed by the patient several years ago. At that time, the patient indicated "Do Not Intubate," "Okay for CPR," "Okay for artificial nutrition," and "No Dialysis." The patient's listed healthcare proxy on the POLST is his son who lives out of state.

Initial ED vital signs are T 102F, HR 120, BP 100/70, RR 25, and SpO_2 88% on 100% O_2 nonrebreather. The patient has dry mucous membranes, coarse breath sounds, and bibasilar crackles. Chest X-ray demonstrates diffuse bilateral patchy infiltrates. Labs are notable for sodium 120, potassium 9, creatinine 2.5 (baseline 0.8), WBC 22 with left-shift, and ABG consistent with severe ARDS (acute respiratory distress syndrome). EKG shows widened QRS and large-peaked T-waves. Bedside ultrasound shows grossly decreased cardiac squeeze with bilateral pulmonary edema and pleural effusions concerning for heart failure.

You recognize that the patient is critically ill and has an ambiguous POLST. For example, it approves CPR, but not intubation, which is an essential part of CPR. You initiate temporizing measures with BiPAP, furosemide, and call the patient's son.

J. K. Bowman (✉)
Department of Emergency Medicine, Massachusetts General Hospital, Boston, MA, USA

Department of Emergency Medicine, Harvard Medical School, Boston, MA, USA

Department of Emergency Medicine, Brigham and Women's Hospital, Boston, MA, USA
e-mail: Jason.Bowman@mgh.harvard.edu

K. Ouchi
Department of Emergency Medicine, Harvard Medical School, Boston, MA, USA

Department of Emergency Medicine, Brigham and Women's Hospital, Boston, MA, USA

© Springer Nature Switzerland AG 2020
K. Aberger, D. Wang (eds.), *Palliative Skills for Frontline Clinicians*,
https://doi.org/10.1007/978-3-030-44414-3_3

Although he recalls his father completing the POLST several years ago, they have not regularly been in touch since. He sounds shocked to hear about his father's current condition, exclaiming: "But he was doing great when I visited him last time!" He also notes that the patient's memory care facility did report concerns about reduced appetite, and there had been some mention of a feeding tube. It will take him several hours to drive to the hospital, and he implores you to "do everything possible" for his father.

Standard Approach

You inform the patient's son of the necessity for emergent intubation, central venous and arterial lines, vasopressors, and emergent dialysis. Given his critical condition and possibility of cardiac arrythmia and/or arrest, the patient is made "full code." You assure the son your team will "do everything" they can for his father and agree to talk more once the son arrives.

You order calcium, insulin and dextrose, albuterol, and bicarbonate for his profound hyperkalemia, and the renal team is consulted for possible emergent dialysis. This appears to be a combined pneumonia and ARDS, as well as possible heart failure and early sepsis. You then give him a gentle IV fluids and empiric antibiotics. The patient is intubated and put on a lung protective ventilator protocol. Your team places a dialysis catheter and arterial line. Ultimately, the patient is admitted to the ICU with anticipated initiation of dialysis and ongoing medical management.

Several days later, you follow up on your patient. He has died. Shortly after admission, the son had arrived to find his father's condition worse. Despite this, and attempts by the ICU team to transition the patient to comfort care, the son continued to insist on a "full code." Subsequently, the patient went into cardiac arrest. The ICU team resuscitated the patient for over 90 minutes before calling the time of death. The ICU team and son are left traumatized by the violence of his death.

Palliative Approach

You order calcium, insulin and dextrose, albuterol, and bicarbonate for his profound hyperkalemia. You defer emergent dialysis given the patient's overall prognosis and his POLST reporting "No dialysis." Empiric antibiotics are given.

Rather than invasive ventilation, given the patient's overall prognosis and POLST reporting he did not wish to be intubated, you instead trial high-flow oxygenation. (Nasal BiPAP is another option.) You recall that nasally delivered respiratory support is often better tolerated by dementia patients than either high flow or BiPAP with a mask. His breathing seems more comfortable on the nasal high flow, and his oxygenation improves moderately.

Before calling the patient's son, you pause for a minute to anticipate a challenging conversation, which will likely need to involve some components of managing

Table 3.1 REMAP framework for goals of care conversations

Reframe	*What is your understanding of what the doctors and dementia facility have told you about your dad's health?* If their understanding appears to differ from the clinical realities, as in this case, consider a follow-up statement such as, *Unfortunately, we're in a different place now. Is it okay if we talk more about what we're seeing here at the bedside and what next steps might be for your dad?*
Expect emotion	Stop talking and listen! Consider responding to emotion directly. Examples of this include, *I can see you're really concerned about this. Is it okay if we talk a bit more about what this means for your dad?* or *I can't imagine what it's been like to hear all this news.* Don't be afraid of silence. The son's impression of his dad is a lot different than what you're telling him now, so this will likely be a large emotional shock.
Map out the future	Try to identify the patient's goals before making any recommendations. For example, you could ask the son, *Given what we've just discussed about the illnesses your dad is dealing with right now, what do you think would be most important to him right now?* or *Thinking about what your dad put in his POLST form, any discussions you've had with him, and your knowledge of him as his son, do you think there are situations or things that he would want to avoid? What would his reasons be for making these decisions? What values in life were most important to him?*
Align with values	*Now that I have a better understanding of what's important to your dad, let's talk a bit more about the options for treatment.*
Propose a plan	It is often helpful to give specific recommendations, rather than simply a list of options. *From what you've told me about what's most important to your dad, I recommend... "How does that sound to you?"*

expected emotions, information gathering, clarifying values and preferences, and making a recommendation. You recall that there are numerous validated tools to help clinicians guide patients and their family/loved ones through difficult conversations. One example of these is the REMAP tool [1], which you quickly pull up on your computer and review (Table 3.1).

In your conversation with the son, he exclaims: "But he was doing great when I visited him last time!" you now recognize the surprise and fear in his voice. You gently explain that the patient likely was doing okay then, but unfortunately he is at a different place now. You ask his permission to talk more about how his father is doing tonight, and briefly describe your evaluation and concerns. After this, you pause and give the son time to process what you've said and try to support him as best you can. You then gently point out that his father had filled out a POLST form. Based on this form, you ask what intervention(s) the son thinks his father would want to avoid.

Box 3.1 Make a Recommendation

It is helpful for many patients and surrogates for the physician to make an informed recommendation after taking time to learn about the patient's wishes and values. Sometimes they appreciate being "given permission" to pursue less aggressive care.

As you are talking with the son, you better understand his perspective and emotion state. You have also helped him identify and focus on his father's stated goals and preferences. You now attempt to align with the father's values with specific informed recommendations based on his current clinical condition:

- Provide a warning shot (e.g., "I'm afraid I have to share a disappointing news") that the patient is critically ill and even with optimal medical management, his risk of dying is high.
- Admit for treatment of pneumonia, acute kidney injury, and electrolyte disturbances.
- Respect foremost the patient's wishes throughout this process, which have been clearly indicated to avoid invasive interventions such as intubation and dialysis.
- Reinforce that comfort will always be a priority as well, and care will also include intensively addressing symptoms such as shortness of breath or agitation (e.g., "I recommend intensive care to relieve his suffering").
- Assure the son that promoting comfort would also indicate foregoing interventions that may cause distress and not yield significant benefit, such as resuscitation, intubation, and dialysis (e.g., I would recommend against CPR or intubation because they are unlikely to help achieve his goals and will cause more suffering).

Box 3.2 Become Emotionally Intelligent
Many statements and questions made by patients and surrogates during goals of care conversations may seem cognitive, perhaps even asking a technical question, but the motivation behind them is emotional – e.g., fear, grief, or guilt. Responding to emotional statements with a purely cognitive answer can cause harm. This is a critically important skill that is often applied poorly, if at all.

You listen carefully to what statements or questions the son offers, considering whether they are cognitive or emotional, and respond in kind. Very few patients and surrogates base goals of care decisions on logic alone, and fewer still have the medical literacy and composure to process technical information in the moment. A technical question may be an unintentional diversion to avoid a concealed moment of fear or grief. Naming the emotion behind the question can get to the root of their fear or guilt (Table 3.2).

After allowing a few moments for reflection, the son agrees that your recommendations best reflect what his father would want. He is on his way to the hospital from out of state, but other family members will soon be there. You affirm this plan, and reassure him that you and your team will continue to closely monitor the patient and provide intensive care and support focused on the goals discussed.

Table 3.2 Emotional versus cognitive responses

But he was doing great when I visited him last time!	Cognitive	*Unfortunately, he is now in combined septic and cardiac shock, and is dying.*
	Emotional	*I can't imagine how much of a surprise this must be for you, then. Unfortunately, your dad is really sick. He has a very serious infection and his heart is failing. We all are with you in hoping for a different outcome, but I worry that he is dying.*
Do everything possible!	Cognitive	*Okay, we'll do CPR, intubation, dialysis, or any other procedures as needed.*
	Emotional	*I hear you, and we will provide your dad with the best care. It sounds like this has been a hard journey, and this now is a scary time. Can I ask you, has your father ever imagined his health worsening to what we see now?*
"I think Dad needs a feeding tube for better nutrition and to get stronger.	Cognitive	*We know from research studies that feeding tubes do not improve functional status, nor decrease the likelihood of aspiration. They lead to discomfort in the abdomen, swelling, and potential complications with the tube itself.*
	Emotional	*Many people, including my own family, think of food as love. We think it is inhumane to withhold food from people we love. But your father's body is shutting down from his illness and he doesn't feel hunger like you and me. Artificial nutrition is not the same as food and will not give him strength. A feeding tube in the stomach may even deprive him of the joy of tasting his favorite foods. Can I talk instead about ways we can increase his comfort?*
So you want to stop/withdrawal care?	Cognitive	*We don't recommend any invasive procedures such as chest compressions or a breathing tube, because they won't help your dad, and will further harm him.*
	Emotional	*I hear your concern. It may feel like we are making a difficult decision, but really it his body that has made this decision today. He is dying a natural death from his illness. I would like to focus on how we can help this process be as comfortable for him as possible, and perhaps that is what he also wished for himself. Knowing him so intimately, what are ways you suggest that we can best attend to his comfort at this time?*

Before moving onto your next patient, you quickly jot down a few critical notes. Incorporating prompts into your EMR and order sets will streamline this process.

Box 3.3 Post Goals of Care Discussion To-Do's
- Update code status orders as needed.
- Once family/loved ones arrive, inquire if there is any additional support that would be important to the patient and/or them, such as a priest or chaplain, or social worker.
- If available in your electronic health record, document your conversation with patient/family/proxy in an easily accessed format, such as a "goals of care" note separate from your ED note.

- Summarize your conversation to the inpatient medical team, ensuring support of the decisions made without reapproaching the conversation from scratch. This provides inpatient teams a starting point for continued discussions. If the goals have been discussed to completion, encourage the inpatient team not to readdress code status or goals so as to avoid causing trauma or guilt/doubt for families.

The patient is admitted to the hospital's intensive care unit to allow for closer monitoring and support. With nasal high-flow oxygenation, titrated low-dose opioids to treat air-hunger, and titrated anxiolytics, the team is able to keep the patient's respiratory rate calm (under 30 breaths per minute), and he appears significantly more comfortable and relaxed. The ICU team turns off all monitors and alarms to help the family focus on the patient and not data, and continues to monitor the patient's vitals from the nurses' station, as well as frequently reassess him.

Over the next several hours, the patient's family and his son/HCP all arrive. A hospital chaplain and social worker each visit and offer support. The family is able to spend several hours talking to the patient, sharing stories with each other about his life. In the early morning hours, the patient's respiratory rate slows, and just before sunrise, he dies peacefully.

Take-Away Points
1. Consider using a validated tool/talking map to help guide conversations with patients and surrogates.
2. Patient's wishes, surrogate wishes, and preferences listed on a POLST often conflict. Whenever possible, even with complex and critically ill patients, take time to try and discern the patient's goals/wishes/priorities and those of their family/health-care surrogates.
3. Strongly consider making a specific recommendation based on your medical expertise and what you've learned from the patient and surrogates about their goals.
4. Emphasize respecting the patient's wishes and goals. Focus on what your team will be doing – treating potentially reversible illness, intensive symptom management, rather than what they will not be doing – not intubating, avoiding CPR.

Reference

1. Childers JW, et al. REMAP: a framework for goals of care conversations. J Oncol Pract. 2017;13(10):e844–50.

Chapter 4
Treating Pain and Prognosticating in Metastatic Cancer

Audrey Tan

Case Introduction

A 64-year-old woman with metastatic lung cancer to the spine, newly diagnosed 2 months prior, presents with back pain to the ED. She is currently undergoing treatment with cisplatin and paclitaxel. Three days prior, she had gradual worsening of pain in the low back after a minor mechanical fall onto the carpet in her house. Yesterday, she took four doses of oxycodone 5 mg by mouth. Early this morning, she took two of the 5 mg tablets together and had moderate relief of her pain for a couple of hours. Her pain is now debilitating and she cannot ambulate.

In the ED, her BP is 130/89, HR 97, O_2 sat 97%, temp 98. On exam, she is awake, in mild distress, with focal tenderness in the right paraspinal lumbar region, mild midline tenderness, intact motor and sensory exams, and no evidence of urinary retention. A non-contrast CT shows a lesion in the L1 vertebral body, which had been present on previous imaging, with no other acute findings.

Usual Approach

Initially, the patient is given acetaminophen as analgesia. Two hours later, she continues to report severe pain. Oral diazepam and IM ketorolac are then given with only minor relief.

An IV is finally started, and she is given 2 mg IV morphine. After no relief, she is admitted for intractable pain, and she continues to receive small doses of morphine IV 6 hours apart, with minimal improvement of symptoms. She is discharged

A. Tan (✉)
Ronald O. Perelman Department of Emergency Medicine, Department of Internal Medicine, New York University School of Medicine, New York, NY, USA
e-mail: audrey.tan@nyulangone.org

© Springer Nature Switzerland AG 2020
K. Aberger, D. Wang (eds.), *Palliative Skills for Frontline Clinicians*,
https://doi.org/10.1007/978-3-030-44414-3_4

with home physical therapy referral, no opioid medications, and follow-up with oncology and her primary care physician.

Palliative Approach

You consider her total opioid usage to determine if she is opioid-naïve or opioid tolerant. She used 20 mg oxycodone yesterday, which is approximately 25 mg oral morphine equivalent (OME). Because she used less than 60 mg OME in the past 24 hours, she is still considered opioid-naïve (Table 4.1).

You decide to give 4 mg morphine IV. You also feel reassured that this is a conservative dose, because she tolerated 10 mg oxycodone this morning, which is equivalent to approximately morphine 5 mg IV. You decide on morphine 4 mg IV after accounting for a 25% dose reduction for cross-tolerance, given that slightly different opioids have different pharmacokinetic profiles (Table 4.2).

You reevaluate her again 15 minutes later, and her pain has only minimally improved. You give a second dose of IV morphine but increase the dose to 6 mg. Fifteen minutes later, her pain has improved to 6/10. After 15 minutes, You administer another dose of 6 mg IV morphine and the pain decreases to 3/10 shortly thereafter. Her pain crisis has been addressed. You discuss with the patient a short admission for continued management of her pain and to establish a new baseline, but she strongly prefers to go home. She ambulates now without difficulty and does not have any signs of respiratory or mental status compromise.

You call her oncologist and recommend a follow-up with the palliative care clinic for symptom management (pain, constipation, psychosocial support). You call the palliative care team, and they request that you bridge her with a 5-day opioid prescription reflecting her current needs, until her first clinic appointment.

Table 4.1 Opioid equianalgesic dosing conversions

Opioid	Parenteral (mg)	Oral (mg)
Morphine	10	25
Hydrocodone	–	25
Hydromorphone	2	5
Oxycodone	–	20
Fentanyl	0.15	–

McPherson ML. Demystifying opioid conversion calculations: a guide for effective dosing. 2nd ed. Bethesda: ASHP; 2018

Table 4.2 Initiating opioids – opioid-naïve patients

	Opioid-naïve	Opioid-tolerant (≥60 OME/day)
Starting dose	Morphine IV 2–5 mg (if no renal impairment)	10–20% of 24 hour usage
Reassess interval	15 minutes to peak IV effect	
Dose escalation	If pain decreased to moderate: Repeat same dose If pain still severe: Increase dose by 50–100%	

Considering her total ED usage of 16 mg morphine IV for this breakthrough pain, you convert this to 40 mg OME. Rounding down to the nearest size tablet, you instruct her to take one morphine sulfate instant release 30 mg tablet every 4 hours as needed. If her pain is only moderate, she can cut the tablet in half, which is safe as it is not a long-acting formulation. You are also sure to prescribe her sennokot to prevent opioid-induced constipation.

The patient is discharged home and presents to palliative care clinic 5 days later. She is taking the morphine PO regularly, and is therefore started on long-acting formulation of morphine sulfate, as well as NSAIDs, bisphosphonates, and low-dose glucocorticoids, all of which help with inflammatory bone pain. She is also scheduled for a close follow-up with radiation oncology which will further address her pain.

Usual Approach (Continued)

She presents to the ED 5 months later in septic shock. After radiochemotherapy, surveillance imaging had demonstrated significant disease progression. She has declined quickly and is now dependent on her family's assistance with activities of daily living (ADLs). She has a home health aide stay with her for most of the day. Over the last 2 days, she has developed fever, generalized weakness, and progressive somnolence (Table 4.3).

Table 4.3 Functional assessment and prognosis

Functional status in the setting of cancer is directly related to prognosis. The Karnovsky Index is a common tool used to assess functional ability.		
Cancer patients with a Karnovsky score of <50% have a median survival of 3 months.		
Able to carry on normal activity and to work; no special care needed.	100	Normal no complaints; no evidence of disease
	90	Able to carry on normal activity; minor signs or symptoms of disease.
	80	Normal activity with effort; some signs or symptoms of disease.
Unable to work; able to live at home and care for most personal needs; varying amount of assistance needed	70	Cares for self; unable to carry on normal activity or to do active work.
	60	Requires occasional assistance, but is able to care for most of his personal needs.
	50	Requires considerable assistance and frequent medical care.
Unable to care for self; requires equivalent of institutional or hospital care; disease may be progressing rapidly.	40	Disabled; requires special care and assistance.
	30	Severely disabled; hospital admission is indicated although death not imminent.
	20	Very sick; hospital admission necessary; active supportive treatment necessary.
	10	Moribund; fatal processes progressing rapidly.
	0	Dead

Karnovsky D, Burchenal J. The clinical evaluation of chemotherapeutic agents in cancer. In: Macleod C, editor. Evaluation of Chemotherapeutic Agents. New York: Columbia University Press; 1949. p. 191–205.

In the ED, her vitals signs are: BP 87/62, HR 125, RR 32, temperature 100.8, O_2 sat 97%. She appears cachectic with temporal wasting, sleepy but arousable, tachypneic with clear lungs, and bilateral lower extremity pitting edema. Urinalysis is grossly positive with +nitrites, +WBC, and + bacteria. You start her on broad-spectrum antibiotics, IVF 30 ml/kg and an antipyretic.

Usual Approach

You place a central line for the initiation of pressors and an arterial line for monitoring blood pressure. Despite your interventions, the patient has increased work of breathing and you intubate for impending respiratory failure. You then admit her to the ICU.

Palliative Approach

You hold off on the intubation and instead start peripheral pressors and BiPAP for increased work of breathing as a temporizing measure while you gather more information and explore goals of care. You also page the oncologist to discuss the cancer prognosis prior to meeting with the family.

You recall a previous lecture about the disease trajectory of cancer, especially in the setting of progressively worsening functional status, now complicated by severe infection. You realize that despite any interventions that you may provide, she is likely near death (Table 4.4).

Before you sit with the patient's daughter, the oncologist returns your call. She states that the patient's cancer has rapidly progressed despite an aggressive chemotherapy regimen, and that there are no further beneficial treatment options at this time. The oncologist had shared this with the patient and daughter; however, they were hopeful she might "get stronger" and benefit from new therapies in development. The oncologist agrees that any further treatment would cause harm and that comfort care and hospice are appropriate.

You sit down with the patient's daughter, Violet, and provide a brief medical update of her mother's critical condition and that you have also spoken with her oncologist.

You: "I am worried about your mother's condition."

Violet (crying): "I understand that she is really sick and that the cancer can't be cured. I don't want her to suffer…she's been through so much…but I just don't want to lose her. They talked to us about this, but I'm not ready to say goodbye. She also has family that I know wants to see her."

You: "Can you tell me what would be most important to your mom right now, knowing that her time is limited?"

Table 4.4 Four functional trajectories of life, from diagnosis of illness to death:

Trajectories of dying

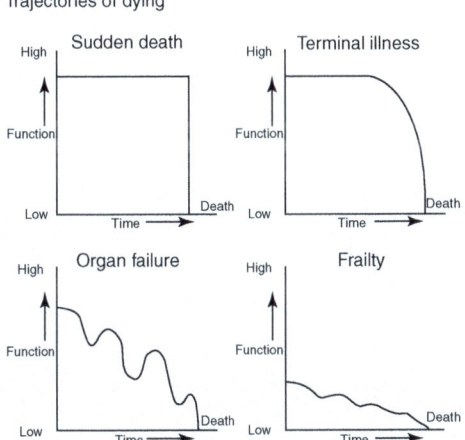

Sudden death: high functional status without significant comorbidity burden that suffers acute survivable insult, e.g., catastrophic myocardial infarction or motor vehicle accident

Terminal illness: maintains high functional status without phenotypic disease burden until final weeks/months when faced with rapid decline (disease "suddenly apparent" or treatment complications), e.g., metastatic solid tumor cancer

Organ failure: recurrent hospitalizations with significant recoveries; however, functional status tends to decrease following each acute care episode resulting in a series of changing baseline functional status episodes until terminal admission, e.g., congestive heart failure, COPD

Frailty: slow progressive functional impairment due to slowly advancing incurable illness, treatable complications often not perceived to be natural part of dying from illness, e.g., advanced dementia, neuromuscular disease

Lunney JR, Lynn J, Hogan C. Profiles of older medicare descendents. J Am Geriatr Soc. 2002; 50: 1108–12.

Violet: "She wouldn't want any of this. She's really independent. She loves to cook and her grandkids. She has always hated hospitals."

You (gently): "Violet, based on what you're telling me, and what I see of her clinical condition, I think that she is dying. It would be a good idea to call family to come as soon as they can. We will continue to support her with the current treatments until they get here. When they arrive, I recommend that we then fully focus on your mother's comfort as our top priority. We may ask another team, palliative care, to support you and your family as well."

Violet: "Ok."

You: "Also based on what we know is happening to her body, I recommend that when your mother's heart stops and she dies, we allow her a natural death and avoid any measures such as an attempt at resuscitation or intubation that may cause her more harm."

Violet: "Yes I agree with that."

You admit the patient to the hospital, place a do-not-resuscitate and do-not-intubate (DNR/DNI) order, place a palliative care consult, and inform the admitting team that the plan for her care is to continue existing interventions with no plans for escalation and a transition to comfort care once the family arrives. Family arrives over the next 24 hours. The patient becomes progressively more obtunded. Palliative care team manages her dyspnea, pain, and agitation, and 2 days later, she dies comfortably.

Take-Away Points
1. Palliative care can help at all stages of disease in patients with serious illness. Early in the course, palliative care provides support and aggressive symptom management to manage pain and potential side effects of disease-directed treatments. Later in the disease course, palliative care continues to provide symptom management in addition to assisting with discussions around goals of care, coordination of care and transitions to hospice at the end of life.
2. ED providers will benefit from having a general understanding of prognosis of various disease states to better guide patients toward appropriate interventions and services.
3. Goals of care conversations are challenging. It is helpful to store some key phrases in your "back pocket." For example, the phrase "I worry…" relays concern about the patient's current critical status, empathy for the patient and loved ones and often serves as a point of transition to the topic of goals of care.
4. At the conclusion of the discussion, remember to provide your patient and family with a recommendation(s) regarding next steps in care, based on their values and the current clinical scenario. Your patients and families will appreciate the guidance that you can provide during these difficult times.

Chapter 5
Complex Pain Management and Goals of Care in a Debilitated Cancer Patient

Marynell Jelinek

Case Introduction

Pearl is a 55-year-old female with metastatic gastric adenocarcinoma, s/p subtotal gastrectomy with a Roux-en-Y gastrojejunostomy. She was discharged to a nursing facility 24 hours ago after a prolonged hospitalization. She was newly diagnosed with her malignancy, and underwent surgical resection with a complicated postoperative course. The oncology team informed her the cancer is incurable, but they suggested palliative chemotherapy once her functional status improves. Prior to that hospitalization, she was taking care of herself, her home, and often her grandchildren. She was discharged to a skilled nursing facility after 11 weeks with a Peripherally Inserted Central Catheter (PICC) line for Total Parenteral Nutrition (TPN), still unable to tolerate adequate fluids and nutrition orally. She was prescribed 15 mg IR (Immediate Release) morphine tablets and ondansetron 8 mg oral tablets upon discharge.

Twenty-four hours later, she presents back to your ED with 8/10 abdominal pain and frequent vomiting. She has tried taking the prescribed morphine, but often vomits immediately after taking it. When she can tolerate the morphine, it reduces the pain to 5/10, but the relief lasts only an hour. She has been unable to transfer out of bed. She is in distress and also frustrated that she had to come back to the hospital.

Usual Approach

You start an IV, give a normal saline fluid bolus, intravenous ondansetron, intravenous analgesic, and consider ordering another CT scan. You order ketorolac 15 mg IV and morphine 2 mg IV, as this is the lowest dose suggested by the order template.

M. Jelinek (✉)
Department of Emergency Medicine, USC Keck School of Medicine,
LAC+USC Medical Center, Los Angeles, CA, USA

© Springer Nature Switzerland AG 2020
K. Aberger, D. Wang (eds.), *Palliative Skills for Frontline Clinicians*,
https://doi.org/10.1007/978-3-030-44414-3_5

Pearl has some pain relief but is still uncomfortable. Shortly after receiving her first dose of morphine, she sends her son to ask for more medication, but the ED is very busy, and it takes almost 2 hours for her to get a second bolus of morphine ordered and delivered. The patient and her son are upset. The expedient disposition plan is to readmit Pearl for intractable pain and further evaluation. She is a "bounceback" to the inpatient team that discharged her just 24 hours ago. Although the patient does not want to be readmitted, she agrees to the plan because she is afraid to go home with her current level of discomfort.

Palliative Approach

From your conversation with the patient and son, you know Pearl has been pre-scribed oral morphine 15 mg, so she can easily tolerate at least a 5 mg dose (3:1 conversion) of parenteral morphine. You also know this dose provided only partial relief, so it is likely she will need a higher dose. You take a few minutes to review her EMR and find she was given hydromorphone 1 mg IV as needed six times dur-ing the 24 hours prior to her discharge. Based on this information, you order hydro-morphone 1 mg IV instead of the usual low-dose morphine suggested by your template.

> **Box 5.1 Malignant Pain Is Treated Differently Than Chronic Nonmalignant Pain**
> In today's climate of opioid crisis and prescription monitoring, many ED phy-sicians are reluctant to use opioids for pain control. We are cautioned not to prescribe opioids because of the risk of overdose, diversion, and addiction. However, the Centers for Disease Control and Prevention have clarified that their opioid use guidelines clearly distinguish cancer-related pain from pre-cautions with generalized chronic pain [1].

Although you generally start with the lowest effective dose, Pearl is likely to have a higher threshold than a patient that is opioid "naïve." She appears small and frail, but has become more tolerant after receiving parenteral opioids several times a day while hospitalized. Because she uses more than 60 mg oral morphine equivalents in the past 24 hours, she is considered opioid tolerant. It is important to get the dose right the first time, knowing delays are inevitable in the ED, which prolong the patient's suffering if you have to order repeated boluses of medication.

Cancer pain is intense and complex, often with both a neuropathic component and central sensitization. A "wind-up" phenomenon can occur where repeated nerve stimulation at CNS pain centers leads to pain from even minimal stimulus (hyperal-gesia), or stimuli that ordinarily do not induce pain (allodynia). Furthermore, opioid use itself can predispose to paradoxical states of hyperalgesia and allodynia. For multiple reasons, pain intensity escalates quickly in patients like Pearl.

Box 5.2 Consider Ketamine as Adjunct Analgesia in Opioid-Refractory Cancer Pain

Parenteral ketamine is a fast-acting adjunct that can be very effective in enhancing pain control in patients with neuropathic pain and/or central sensitization. Ketamine targets NMDA receptors and can often disrupt the pain cycle. It also potentiates the analgesic strength of opioids. Benefits may persist for up to weeks following even a one-time ED dose.

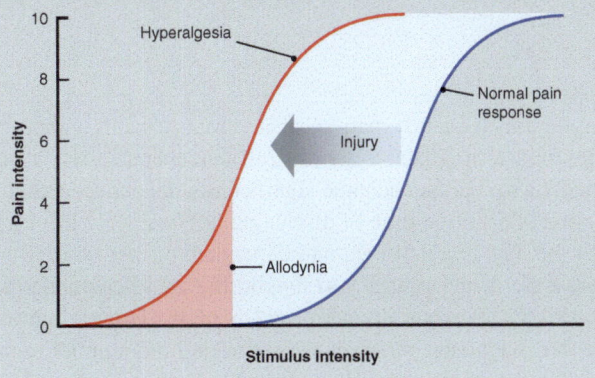

The patient's PICC line is accessed so as to avoid another venipuncture. She is given hydromorphone 1 mg IV. After 15 minutes, her pain has only improved minimally, and you administer a second dose of 1 mg hydromorphone. When you reassess her, she is still grimacing and reports her pain as moderate. She appears to be slightly sleepy. At this point, you trial ketamine 0.3 mg/kg slow IV push (alternatively diluted in 100 ml infused over 15 minutes). Following this, she is more comfortable; however, given her recent hurried discharge and significant ED analgesic needs, you believe she might benefit from a brief admission to determine a stable long-acting analgesia regimen.

It is now important to consider the patient's goals at the present moment, not just the disposition decision. You acknowledge her wish to avoid hospitalization, but help her recognize it will not be comfortable for her at home. You suggest that she will benefit from a long-acting medication, either orally or through a patch (e.g., fentanyl), which will improve her quality of life and allow her to be more functionally independent. Because it will take up to 2–3 days for these medications to reach steady state, you suggest she remain in the hospital to receive relief through short-acting oral/parenteral opioids in order to prevent a reoccurrence of a pain crisis. You recommend a palliative care consult to manage this medication transition. She appreciates your thoughtfulness and agrees to stay.

Table 5.1 Poorer Functional Outcomes After Chemotherapy [2]

Patients with ECOG ≥3 have not been to shown to significantly benefit from further chemotherapy. Some studies demonstrate that patients with ECOG ≥2 receiving chemotherapy in the final months of life experience worse quality of life without increased overall survival [3].

ECOG	Description
0	Fully active, able to carry on all pre-disease performance without restriction.
1	Restricted in physically strenuous activity but ambulatory and able to carry out work of a light or sedentary nature, e.g., light house work, office work.
2	Ambulatory and capable of all selfcare but unable to carry out any work activities. Up and about more than 50% of waking hours.
3	Capable of only limited selfcare, confined to bed or chair more than 50% of waking hours.
4	Completely disabled. Cannot carry on selfcare. Totally confined to bed or chair.
5	Dead

You also pause to consider the patient's performance status and prognosis as they may dictate her long-term goals. Pearl was fully independent when she entered the hospital 3 months ago, but has become significantly deconditioned during her prolonged hospitalization. At the time of discharge, her quality of life was poor. She is in bed most of the day, unable to eat and dependent on her family for most of her self-care. There is no strong evidence to support the use of chemotherapy for cancer patients with ECOG (Eastern Cooperative Oncology Group) scores of three or greater. Given her diagnosis, performance status and the number of complications she has endured, her performance status is not likely to improve and chemotherapy would likely be harmful (Table 5.1).

Because her treatment options are limited, you broach a discussion with her about her goals of care. You gently ask her, "What would be important to you if your time were short?" She is startled at the direct question, but also deeply appreciates your willingness to discuss an issue that she has thus far avoided. She has felt like she is declining for a while and agrees that she would not tolerate treatment. She just wants to return home and be with her family.

With that primary goal in mind, you introduce hospice as an additional layer of support, a comprehensive team that now brings care to her. They deliver medications, equipment, medical, social, spiritual, and nursing care to optimize comfort for her remaining life. Pain and other symptoms can be closely monitored and controlled. As symptoms worsen, hospice care will intensify. They can be with her several hours continuously a day and are always accessible 24/7. Hospice would strive to prevent pain crises and allow her to maximize her time at home.

Pearl recalls hearing about hospice from her friends. She asks: "Am I giving up?" You reassure her that her decision reflects her acceptance of what is happening in her body and her wish to enjoy fully whatever time is left. Furthermore, should her health improve, she can revoke hospice services at any time to pursue disease-focused treatments. Seeing her process so much information already, you decide to forego discussion of code status for now, given she remains clinically stable. Patients enrolled in hospice are not required to be DNR/DNI.

> **Box 5.3 Hospice Does Not Equate to DNR Code Status**
> There is no mandated code status for hospice enrollment. A significant portion of hospice patients are full code when they enroll. Code status conversations continue with hospice social workers and nurses as the patients' disease and quality of life evolve. Many patients and families who are reluctant to consider the finality of code status usually need time to process their emotions. Forcing a decision about code status after an already difficult decision about hospice care may sometimes cause more harm than benefit.

Pearl is admitted and the palliative team establishes an effective combination of long-acting and short-acting opiates to control her pain. Your initial ED conversations provided ample time for her and her family to consider these important decisions. The admitting hospitalist was initially surprised that you discussed hospice with this patient. However, upon further reflection, she agrees with your intervention. You also update Pearl's oncologist, who appreciates your initiative with her. She had been unable to approach this topic in the past given the patient's reluctance and unwavering optimism.

Following admission, the palliative care team continues the hospice conversation. Hospice will not usually continue TPN, and this becomes a key issue. Even though Pearl accepts that it will not improve her functionality, her family is fearful that she may die from hunger. Ultimately, she is discharged home with home health and ongoing TPN nutritional support. She becomes increasingly somnolent over the next 2 weeks and is enrolled onto hospice. TPN is then stopped, as it no longer provides benefit. Her family is encouraged to give her small tastes of her favorite foods. Two weeks later, she dies.

> **Take-Away Points**
> 1. Larger doses of opioids are required for patients with malignant pain, who have developed opioid tolerance.
> 2. Consider ketamine as adjunct analgesia in opioid-refractory cancer pain.
> 3. Although often pursued, palliative chemotherapy in advanced cancer patients with poor functional status and prognoses of weeks to months is not helpful and may significantly worsen symptom burden.
> 4. Hospice patients are not required to have DNR code status.

References

1. Dowell D, et al. No shortcuts to safer opioid prescribing. N Engl J Med. 2019;380(24):2285–7.
2. Oken M, Creech R, Tormey D, et al. Toxicity and response criteria of the Eastern Cooperative Oncology Group. Am J Clin Oncol. 1982;5:649–55.
3. Prigerson HG, et al. Chemotherapy use, performance status, and quality of life at the end of life. JAMA Oncol. 2015;1(6):778–84.

Chapter 6
To Intubate or Not to Intubate: Asking the Right Questions

Nitin Ubhayakar

Case Introduction

EMS transports a 96-year-old female in respiratory distress from a local nursing facility to the ED. She has a history of dementia, hypertension, and hyperlipidemia. The nursing facility staff called 911 this morning after finding the patient tachycardic, tachypneic, and hypoxic. At baseline, she is alert and oriented to person only.

On arrival to the ED, her vital signs are: T 101.2F, HR 136, RR 36, and SpO_2 86% on a nonrebreather, but she remains normotensive. Physical exam reveals a cachectic, frail-looking female, with temporal wasting, in obvious respiratory distress. She has coarse breath sounds most notably in the right lung fields. Although her eyes open intermittently, she is unable to follow commands. Multiple decubitus ulcers in various stages are also appreciated on skin examination. The patient's blood sugar is 128.

She is placed on a monitor, IV access is established, and you order appropriate labs, including blood cultures. Stat portable X-ray reveals a right middle-lobe infiltrate, confirming your suspicion of aspiration pneumonia. After reviewing the patient's known allergies, you order an antipyretic, IV fluids, and broad-spectrum antibiotics. Within a few minutes, the patient's family arrives, and you initiate a goals-of-care discussion.

N. Ubhayakar (✉)
Emergency Medicine Physician, White Memorial Hospital, Los Angeles, CA, USA

Palliative Care Physician, Huntington Memorial Hospital, Pasadena, CA, USA

© Springer Nature Switzerland AG 2020
K. Aberger, D. Wang (eds.), *Palliative Skills for Frontline Clinicians*,
https://doi.org/10.1007/978-3-030-44414-3_6

Usual Approach

You begin by explaining the patient's clinical condition and express your concerns regarding her tenuous respiratory status: "She is having difficulty breathing due to pneumonia." You then discuss treatment options: "Since she is having trouble breathing, I could put in a breathing tube to help her breathe." You also discuss code status: "Given how sick she is, if her heart were to stop, would she want us to do everything we can to bring her back?" The patient's family is emotionally overwhelmed and unable to make decisions. She is eventually intubated and admitted to the ICU for ongoing medical management. The patient has a prolonged ICU course and is unable to be weaned from the ventilator. Her family consents to tracheostomy and gastrostomy tubes, and she is later discharged to a long-term care facility.

> **Box 6.1 No Such Thing as Impartiality**
> As the physician, you know what treatment options are available, and what functional outcomes may or may not be achieved by these interventions. It is imperative to guide the family by making recommendations based on what you know about the patient, rather than giving them a menu of options. The words you choose, how you say them, or even the absence of a thorough conversation – all may introduce bias. Even families with high medical literacy sometimes make decisions not based on logic, but their emotional state during a highly stressful time. Remember: Although physicians want to talk about treatments, patients/families want to talk about outcomes.

Palliative Approach

Given the patient's increased work of breathing and hypoxia, you use NPPV or noninvasive positive pressure ventilation (e.g., high-flow nasal cannula or BiPAP) as a temporizing measure to improve the patient's respiratory parameters. You then have a discussion with the patient's family.

You ask about the patient's overall health, and the quality of her daily life. You learn that she has been hospitalized with increasing frequency over the last year. This is her third ED visit in 6 months. You ask if the patient had completed any advance care planning: "Has she ever made her last wishes known?" "What outcome is the family hoping for now?" You learn that the family has seen her quality of life waning; she can no longer appreciate gardening or tolerate visits from her grandchildren. Before dementia and her functional decline, she was a spirited woman who made her own decisions and lived independently (Table 6.1).

Table 6.1 5-minute goals-of-care framework

Minutes 1–2	Elicit patient understanding of underlying illness and today's acute change. If available, build off previous advance directives or documented conversations. Acquire a sense of patient's values and desired quality of life (to help frame prognosis and priorities for interventions). Name and validate observed goals, hopes, fears, and expectations.
Minutes 3–4	Discuss treatment options using reflected language, and focusing on functional outcomes. Continually re-center on patient's (not family's) wishes and values. Recommend a course of action, avoiding impartiality when prognosis is dire.
Minute 5	Summarize and discuss next steps. Introduce appropriate ancillary ED resources (e.g., hospice/observation unit, social work, chaplain).

Adapted from Wang [1]

You then update the family on the patient's current medical condition: "She is having breathing difficulties due to pneumonia, which is common in the final stages of dementia." Her family is not surprised to hear this, especially after discussing her recent downward trajectory. What the family has shared with you about the patient now guides your treatment recommendations: "Given what you have told me about your mother, it makes sense to continue doing what we are doing now hoping she will overcome the infection. However, if her body shows further signs of weakening, I suggest we recognize that she is dying and at that point, not perform CPR, or put her on life support. Instead we would focus on keeping her comfortable, and allow a natural death." The family agrees as they believe this honors her character.

You call the hospitalist, and before she meets the family, you discuss all that has ensued with this patient and her family. She agrees with your plan and subsequently reinforces it with the family, i.e., she will continue noninvasive ventilation and antibiotics, but not escalate care further. Speaking with the consultant(s) (e.g., primary team, critical care, other specialists) prior to their communication with family regarding your goals-of-care conversation can help to avoid confusion that occurs when other providers attempt to have similar discussions. It can also strengthen a patient's/family's decision to avoid aggressive interventions such as intubation and resuscitation in situations where it may not provide benefit (Table 6.2).

The patient is admitted to the medical floor with the pulmonology team as consultants. As needed medications are made available to address the patient's symptoms including dyspnea. Despite IV antibiotics and NPPV, her clinical condition continues to decline. On hospital day three, the family meets with the hospitalist, and the decision is made to transition the patient to comfort care. She is compassionately weaned from NPPV, and a few hours later, dies peacefully with her family at bedside.

Table 6.2 Word choice matters in goals-of-care conversations

Avoid these phrases	Consider these phrases
We need to discuss code status.	Tell me about your mother.
I wouldn't want this for my own mother.	What was she like before she became ill? How has this illness affected her quality of life?
I don't believe resuscitation would be successful. It is highly unlikely that she would ever get off these life-support machines.	It seems like this illness has already taken much of her. From what I see today, I do not think she would be able to return to a quality of life that was meaningful to her. This is the natural course of her disease, and she is now dying.
Do you want us to do everything? Would she want heroic measures? Do you want us to push on her chest or put a breathing tube down her throat?	Based on what you have told me about your mother, do you think she would want to die a natural death?
There is nothing more we can do.	I wish things were different. I suggest that we shift our focus now to keeping her comfortable, and aggressively use medications to reduce any distress she may feel.

Adapted from Wang [2]

Take-Away Points

1. Do not offer or perform an intervention if you do not feel it will benefit the patient. (See ACEP's policy on "Nonbeneficial ("Futile") Emergency Medical Interventions) [3].
2. If possible, consider non-invasive interventions like high flow nasal cannula or bipap in patients who are unlikely to benefit from endotracheal intubation.
3. ED goals-of-care conversations should frame treatment options in terms of patient's prior quality of life and desired outcomes. Not asking these questions leads to medical decision-making that may not achieve true informed consent.
4. Approach goals-of-care conversations like any other procedure. Refine your technique through practice of careful word choice and timing.

References

1. Wang DH. Beyond code status: palliative care begins in the emergency department. Ann Emerg Med. 2017;69(4):437–43. https://doi.org/10.1016/j.annemergmed.2016.10.027.
2. Wang D, Creel-Bulos C. A systematic approach to comfort care transitions in the emergency department. J Emerg Med. 2019;56(3):267–74. https://doi.org/10.1016/j.jemermed.2018.10.027.
3. Simon JR, Kraus C, Rosenberg M, Wang DH, Clayborne EP, Derse AR. 'Futile Care'-An emergency medicine approach: ethical and legal considerations. Ann Emerg Med. 2017;70(5):707–13.

Chapter 7
ED Approach to the Hospice Patient

Monique Schaulis

Case Introduction

A 66-year-old man on hospice for metastatic lung cancer is brought into the ED via 911 for fever and cough for the last 2 days. Medics report that his caregiver was concerned the patient was somewhat confused and he called 911. They report a language barrier, so they are not 100% sure what is going on. They found a POLST (Physicians Orders for Life Sustaining Treatment) stating DNR with limited interventions, which was signed 8 months ago as part of his hospice documents. They do not believe caregiver has contacted hospice today. Paramedics attempted, but were unable, to place an IV. From the electronic medical record, you see that he was referred to hospice after his last hospitalization for sepsis 2 weeks ago. Unfortunately, you cannot read the hospice notes in your EMR, so you are not sure what has happened since then.

Vital signs: BP 90/60, HR 113, RR 28 T 102, sat 93%. The patient's exam demonstrates a cachectic, moderately distressed, disoriented man. He has decreased breath sounds at the right base, however, maintains normal work of breathing. Without any testing, you strongly suspect sepsis secondary to pneumonia in this end-stage lung cancer hospice patient. You know that while it is possible that antibiotics may help the infection temporarily, the patient will die before long, most likely within hours to days. You worry that any disease-focused treatment will be futile and painful.

M. Schaulis (✉)
The Permanente Medical Group, San Francisco, CA, USA

© Springer Nature Switzerland AG 2020
K. Aberger, D. Wang (eds.), *Palliative Skills for Frontline Clinicians*,
https://doi.org/10.1007/978-3-030-44414-3_7

Usual Approach

1. ED workup includes the sepsis bundle with aggressive IV fluids, empiric broad-spectrum antibiotics, and imaging.
2. Admission to hospitalist with oncology consult.
3. Hospitalist may consider palliative consult.

Palliative Approach

1. Attend to patient's distress: O_2 for his increased work of breathing, oral/rectal acetaminophen for his fever, and oral morphine concentrated liquid (20 mg/ml) 5 mg for his restlessness, which you think is from discomfort. You may consider using the IV route, but it may be unnecessary.
2. Call the hospice agency to understand what has been happening with this patient and family. They may know exactly why the patient is in your ED and help you manage this difficult situation.
3. Call family.
4. Empiric antibiotics are not imperative in this situation, but you may consider them. You can discuss this with hospice and family.
5. Consider the viability of a discharge home despite inevitability of death.

Box 7.1 What Is the Role of Antibiotics at the End of Life?

Fifty years ago, many people died "naturally in their sleep." Had they presented to a modern ED, the vast majority would have been readily identified as septic and dehydrated. Infections constitute a natural death, a final common destination from many disease trajectories (e.g., dementia, cancer and other immunocompromised states, neurologic dysfunction.)

Antibiotics may reverse an infection and grant patients more meaningful time. Hospice often utilizes oral antibiotics. These decisions are individual and should be explored with the patient. Consider also the risks of antibiotics, including adverse reactions, diarrhea, and both the physical impact to patient and psychological impact to family of prolonging the dying process.

Compared to the usual approach, in this case, the palliative approach integrates two key principles:

- Attend to patient comfort rather than using standard sepsis protocol. Avoid multiple needle sticks or other procedures that will be distressing. Be sure the patient is clean, the room temperature is comfortable, without a lot of noise. Try to avoid alarming monitors, bright lights, and frequent interruptions.
- Focus on excellent communication with the hospice team, patient, and family. Try to think of the family as your patients as well. Approach conversation with them as a procedure. Your goal is to make them feel their brother is getting excellent care.

Hospice patients presenting to the ED may feel confused or even frustrated. You too may feel conflicted in determining the best treatment options:

1. Should you initiate sepsis workup and treatment?
2. Should the patient be admitted?
3. Is the code status accurate?

Rather than a piecemeal approach, consider using the questions below to determine your diagnosis and disposition of the patient (Table 7.1).

If it appears that the surrogates did not understand the purpose of hospice, or the patient's poor prognosis, you need to step back and conduct a broader goals

Table 7.1 Key questions to understand why the hospice patient came to the ED

Question to ask	Purpose
I understand your loved one is receiving hospice services. What brought you all to the ED today?	Surrogates may identify reason for distress: misunderstanding of hospice services, etc.
How has your experience with hospice been so far?	May clue you in to how expectations have, or have not, been met and what is important.
Were you able to get in touch with hospice before calling 911?	Sometimes families call 911 because it is faster, but sometimes they just do not know that hospice has 24/7 availability.
[If an acute change is mentioned] *What do you understand about what this means for your loved one?*	If needed, gently break bad news about dying and provide reassurance and normalization of signs of dying and associated emotions by surrogates.
How are you and the rest of their support network coping?	911 call may sometimes be a caregiver's emotional response to witnessing the patient's active dying.
If your loved one could see themselves and speak for themselves, what do you think they would say is most important right now? Follow-up: *Have they ever mentioned if they had feelings about dying in the hospital* versus *home?*	Conversation now shifts into decision-making.

Table 7.2 REMAP Framework for Goals-of-Care Conversations

Step	What you say or do
1. Reframe why the status quo isn't working.	You may need to discuss serious news (e.g., a scan result) first. *Given this news, it seems like a good time to talk about what to do now.* *We're in a different place.*
2. Expect emotion and empathize.	*It's hard to deal with all this.* *I can see you are really concerned about [x].* *Tell me more about that—what are you worried about?* *Is it ok for us to talk about what this means?*
3. Map the future.	*Given this situation, what's most important for you?* *When you think about the future, are there things you want to do?* *As you think toward the future, what concerns you?*
4. Align with the patient's values.	*As I listen to you, it sounds the most important things are [x,y,z].*
5. Plan medical treatments that match patient values.	*Here's what I can do now that will help you do those important things. What do you think about this?*

conversation. In these situations, consider using the REMAP talking map to help guide [1, 2] (Table 7.2).

> **Box 7.2 Nobody Wants to "Give Up"**
> When you speak with the family/surrogate, discuss what you've done to make the patient comfortable. This will help demonstrate you care. Tell them what you *have* done before you mention what you would not or cannot do.

Applying the REMAP framework to your conversation with the patient's family:

- Reframe: The serious news now is the patient's time is short, in the range of hours to days. Explain that the current situation is one of the final phases of cancer. You know this because the patient's functional status has declined rapidly and he has had two serious episodes of sepsis in the last few weeks. In the cancer disease trajectory, function often declines quickly in the last month of life.
- Expect Emotion: Despite the fact that this patient is enrolled in hospice, don't assume that the family knows he is dying imminently. You may need to gently break this bad news to them. Normalize the dying process, but be unambiguous by clearly stating "dying." Expect emotion from family and respond with empathy. Communicate verbally and nonverbally that you will support him/them during this difficult time.
- Map the Future: Knowing that he is in the final phase of life, would he want to be home? Are they equipped to take care of him there? What is most important now?

Box 6.3 Sometimes Surrogates Seek Permission, Not Agency
Avoid asking the family "What do you want us to do?" That may lead to a clinically nonbeneficial request. Moreover, sometimes surrogates feel guilty verbalizing, especially in front of others present, a decision for less treatment. Providing a clear recommendation may prevent them feeling they actively abandoned their loved one. Instead, they chose to maximize their loved one's comfort and trusted the doctors' expertise.

Align: "As I listen to you, it sounds like being home and being comfortable are the most important things now."

Plan Medical Treatments to Match Goals: "You have hospice in place already to support him and your family at home. Given that we know he is dying, and we don't want to prolong his suffering, we will treat his symptoms aggressively, but will not start antibiotics. Let's speak with the caregiver again about not calling 911 but rather calling hospice instead. Does that sound about right?"

Code status has already been documented in the POLST. You do not need to readdress it unless there is a specific reason. However, if the patient is to be discharged, you may consider a recommendation for a POLST stating comfort care at this point. You might say, "In this stage it may be best to lean on hospice to maximize his comfort at home rather than facing the frustration of coming back to the hospital."

Take-Away Points
1. It is not necessary to adhere to the usual sepsis protocols for hospice patients. Detailed documentation of patient's goals of care will exempt you from protocols.
2. Give the big picture information to the patient/caregivers clearly and without medical jargon. You may have to break bad news that even though the patient has been on hospice that death is imminent.
3. Communicate with hospice before undertaking the standard workup. They can help you understand the reason for presentation, manage symptoms, communicate with the family, and create a plan for disposition.
4. If the patient has a DNR order, you do not need to readdress code status each time a hospice patient comes to the ED. Repeated code status conversations are emotionally burdensome to families and can make them feel that they are responsible for his death.

References

1. Childers JW, et al. REMAP: a framework for goals of care conversations. J Oncol Pract. 2017;13(10):e844–50.
2. Vital Talk, 2019, https://www.vitaltalk.org/guides/transitionsgoals-of-care/.

Part II
Inpatient Medicine

Chapter 8
I Can't Let Him Starve: Artificial Nutrition in Patients with Advanced Dementia

Emily Jean Martin

Case Introduction

Mr. S is an 87-year-old man with advanced dementia who presents with tachypnea, a productive cough, fever, and somnolence. He lives at home with his daughter, Caroline, who serves as his primary caretaker and medical surrogate. At baseline, Mr. S is bedbound, incontinent of stool and urine, dependent in all activities of daily living, and largely nonverbal. He has been losing weight and requires frequent cueing during meals. Mr. S has been hospitalized three times in the past year, once for aspiration pneumonia and twice for urinary tract infections. Caroline states, "he's had a rough year, but he always bounces back."

Mr. S is admitted to the medicine service with sepsis secondary to aspiration pneumonia. Despite optimal medical management, one week into his hospitalization he remains somnolent and has failed consecutive swallow evaluations. Caroline is frustrated that her father is "wasting away" in the hospital and questions you, "How is he supposed to get better when he's not getting any nutrition?" A nasogastric tube is placed to temporarily provide enteral nutrition. The following day, Mr. S appears more alert, opening his eyes to voice and occasionally mumbling. Caroline attributes his improved mentation to the initiation of enteral nutrition. Within 48 hours, however, he has pulled out the nasogastric tube twice. Other than his lack of enteral nutrition, he is medically stable for discharge. You arrange to meet with Caroline to discuss the plan of care regarding his dysphagia.

E. J. Martin (✉)
Palliative Care Program, Department of Medicine,
UCLA David Geffen School of Medicine, Los Angeles, CA, USA
e-mail: EJMartin@mednet.ucla.edu

© Springer Nature Switzerland AG 2020
K. Aberger, D. Wang (eds.), *Palliative Skills for Frontline Clinicians*,
https://doi.org/10.1007/978-3-030-44414-3_8

Usual Approach

You coordinate with Caroline to round on Mr. S when she will be present. In your charting that morning, you identify "lack of nutrition" as his primary medical problem. His laboratory and diagnostic studies have all been otherwise unactionable.

> **Box 8.1 Aspiration in End-Stage Dementia is Part of the Natural History of Disease and an Expected Trajectory Toward Death**
> Dementia is a terminal neurodegenerative illness. The typical disease trajectory is characterized by gradual, progressive cognitive and functional decline interspersed with episodes of rapid clinical deterioration and incomplete recovery [1–3]. Advanced disease is characterized by profound cognitive deficits, inability to ambulate, incontinence, and oropharyngeal dysphagia often resulting in malnutrition, dehydration, and aspiration pneumonia.

In your meeting with Caroline, you state: "I would like to talk about your father's medical care. As we previously discussed, the use of a nasogastric tube is only a temporary measure. Given that he has pulled it out twice, I don't recommend reinserting it as we would need to put him in restraints. Since he has not passed his swallow study, he still cannot eat safely by mouth. So, now we need to make a decision. Do you want him to have a feeding tube?"

Caroline appears tense and confused. She states adamantly that she wants "everything done" to help her father regain his strength and to receive sufficient nutrition. You interject that placement of a percutaneous feeding tube will not reduce her father's risk of aspiration and that, given his poor prognosis, would not be recommended." Caroline accuses you of "giving up" on her father and yells: "I can't let him starve!"

Following this conversation, a percutaneous endoscopic gastrostomy is performed and artificial nutrition is initiated. Mr. S continues to be somnolent and has periods of acute agitation during which he pulls at his gastric tube and intravenous lines. He requires frequent use of wrist restraints and antipsychotics. Following a prolonged hospital course, he is discharged to a skilled nursing facility despite Caroline's preference to have him at home. He returns to the emergency department three times within the next two months, once for a dislodged feeding tube and twice for aspiration pneumonia. He ultimately dies in the hospital from respiratory failure and septic shock, three months after placement of the gastric tube. Caroline feels helpless having watched her father continue to suffer, never getting stronger as she had hoped.

Box 8.2 Many Decisions for Artificial Nutrition do not Reflect True Informed Consent

Surrogate decision makers for patients with advanced dementia are frequently asked to make decisions regarding initiation of percutaneous enteral nutrition without a clear understanding of the disease trajectory, expected prognosis, or burdens besides the usual risks and benefits [2, 4]. In a mortality follow-back survey of 486 next-of-kin decedents of individuals with dementia, of those who had received a percutaneous feeding tube, 14% reported having no discussion with a health-care provider prior to tube insertion. Of those who reported having a discussion, in 42% of cases the conversation lasted less than 15 minutes, in half there was no discussion of the risks of feeding tube insertion, and in one-third, the option of hand-feeding was not mentioned. Thirty-eight percent of respondents reported that the physician was "strongly in favor" of inserting a percutaneous feeding tube and 11% felt pressured by the physician to proceed with tube placement. Twenty-six percent of respondents stated the feeding tube was inserted to make it easier for staff to feed the patient [5].

Palliative Approach

You meet Caroline at the entrance to Mr. S' hospital room. Since you were unable to reliably obtain any preferences from Mr. S and his presence during this conversation may only distract Caroline from an important discussion, you invite her to talk in a quiet, private room. You confirm with Caroline that no one else needs to be present for this meeting. You outline what you hope to address and invite her to do the same. She explains that her priority is making sure that her father gets sufficient nutrition, as she "can't stand the idea that he is starving."

Box 8.3 Distinguishing Artificial Nutrition from "Food"

Conversations about dementia-associated dysphagia should be person-centered and approached with sensitivity to the emotional and symbolic meaning that many individuals place on food and feeding [6, 7]. While artificial nutrition may lead to weight stabilization and adiposity increase, it does not lead to increased muscle mass or improved functional outcomes.

You acknowledge Caroline's concerns and assure her that you will address them. You ask her to share her understanding of her father's clinical condition. You use open-ended, exploratory questions to learn about his life, including his expressed goals and core values. You ask Caroline what she is most worried about regarding her father's health as well as what she is most hopeful for. As

Caroline recounts both how remarkable her father's life has been and also how much it has changed, you respond with empathic statements. When she begins to cry, you thoughtfully allow for therapeutic silence. You acknowledge what a strong advocate she has been for her father and applaud her efforts to care for him.

During the conversation, Caroline describes Mr. S as a stubborn and fiercely independent man. He had spent much of his life as an avid fisherman, which Caroline characterizes as "more of an obsession than a hobby." He disliked being indoors or in large crowds. More recently, Caroline notes that her father has appeared happiest when sitting on his porch, looking out at the expansive hills past his yard. You thank Caroline for sharing so openly and ask for permission to now shift the focus of the conversation to discussing the next steps in her father's care.

Empathically, you help Caroline reframe her father's condition in terms of the end of life. You describe the progressive functional and cognitive decline punctuated by acute illness that is typical of dementia. You explain his dysphagia and weight loss in terms of his underlying, irreversible neurodegenerative disease, emphasizing the high likelihood of recurrent aspiration pneumonia. You detail the potential risks, benefits, and burdens of percutaneous tube insertion for artificial nutrition. You introduce the alternative option of careful hand-feeding for comfort.

Box 8.4 Discussing the Risks, Benefits, and Alternatives
Based on the available evidence, percutaneous tube feeding in the setting of advanced dementia does not improve survival, quality of life, physical functioning, or nutritional parameters (weight, albumin) nor does it decrease the risk of pressure, ulcers, or aspiration [6, 8, 9]. Further, percutaneous tube feeding may introduce additional harms including the need for physical restraints or sedating medications to reduce the risk of patients pulling the tube out, or the need for additional procedures if the tube is dislodged [5]. Alternatives, including hand-feeding for comfort, should be discussed [10]. Both the American Geriatrics Society and the American Academy of Hospice and Palliative Medicine recommend against artificial nutrition in advanced dementia.

Caroline appears overwhelmed weighing these risks and benefits. You gently ask, "If the healthy Mr. S from years ago could see himself now, knowing that he is nearing the end of his life, what do you think he would say?" Caroline pauses. After a few moments, she looks up. "He'd say, 'Take me home.'" After further discussion about Mr. S' core values and previously expressed priorities, you introduce the role of hospice care in allowing Mr. S to be at home at the end of his life with his care focused on optimizing his comfort. Caroline appreciates that you took the time to learn about her father and that you helped her place him at the center of this decision-making process.

Two days later, Mr. S is discharged home with hospice. Over the next several weeks, he is carefully hand-fed by his daughter and visiting family members. As expected, he develops another aspiration pneumonia. After a discussion with Caroline, the hospice agency starts him on a trial of oral antibiotics at home. The following week, he becomes increasingly somnolent. Antibiotics are discontinued and the patient's symptoms are well palliated until he dies a natural death. Caroline is grateful that her father could spend his remaining days at home.

Take-Away Points
1. Patients/families should be informed that dementia is a progressive, irreversible, terminal illness and that dysphagia, weight loss, recurrent aspiration, and infections are a natural and inevitable result of the underlying disease process.
2. A false dichotomy between tube feeding and strict NPO is often presented to patients/families. Hand-feeding for comfort should be discussed as a viable alternative to artificial nutrition for patients with advanced dementia.
3. Current evidence demonstrates that percutaneous tube feeding in patients with advanced dementia does not improve survival, quality of life, physical functioning, or weight gain, nor does it reduce aspiration risk. It may, however, introduce additional complications and increase patient and caregiver distress.
4. Several national guidelines recommend against percutaneous feeding tubes in advanced dementia.

References

1. Lunney JR, Lynn J, Foley DJ, et al. Patterns of functional decline at the end of life. JAMA. 2003;289(18):2387–92.
2. Mitchell SL, Teno JM, Kiely DK, et al. The clinical course of advanced dementia. N Engl J Med. 2009;361:1529–38.
3. Gill TM, Gahbauer EA, Han L, Allore HG. Trajectories of disability in the last year of life. N Engl J Med. 2010;362:1173–80.
4. Stokes LA, Combes H, Stokes G. Understanding the dementia diagnosis: the impact on the caregiving experience. Dementia. 2014;13(1):59–78.
5. Teno JM, Mitchell SL, Kuo SK. Decision-making and outcomes of feeding tube insertion: a five state study. J Am Geriatr Soc. 2011;59(5):881–6.
6. Sampson EL, Candy B, Jones L. Enteral tube feeding for older people with advanced dementia. Cochrane Database Syst Rev. 2009;2:CD007209.
7. Yamagishi A, Morita T, Miyashita M, et al. The care strategy for families of terminally ill cancer patients who become unable to take nourishment orally: recommendations from a nationwide survey of bereaved family members' experiences. J Pain Symptom Manag. 2010;40(5):671–83.
8. Teno JM, Gozalo PL, Mitchell SL, et al. Does feeding tube insertion and its timing improve survival? J Am Geriatr Soc. 2012;60(10):1918–21.
9. Murphy LM, Lipman TO. Percutaneous endoscopic gastrostomy does not prolong survival in patients with dementia. Arch Intern Med. 2003;163(11):1351–3.
10. Hanson LC. Tube feeding versus assisted oral feeding for persons with dementia: using evidence to support decision-making. Ann Long Term Care Clin Care Aging. 2013;21(1):36–9.

Chapter 9
Shared Decision-Making in the Setting of a Large Ischemic Stroke

Cara Siegel and Jessica Besbris

Case Introduction

A 78-year-old woman with a history of atrial fibrillation, hypertension, and chronic kidney disease was found on the floor this morning by her daughter. On arrival to the ED, she is aphasic and her right side is not moving. She demonstrates absent blink to threat over the right visual field. She is also in atrial fibrillation. Her total NIH stroke scale score is 30. Her blood glucose is 150 mmol/L, and her creatinine is 1.9 μmol/L; other laboratory values are unremarkable. Her imaging reveals an occlusion in the M1 branch of the left middle cerebral artery and a large completed infarction in the corresponding parenchyma in the left hemisphere. She is not a candidate for IV thrombolysis or thrombectomy because of the unknown time from onset of her symptoms and the size of completed infarction on imaging.

The patient is admitted to the intensive care unit for post-acute stroke care, where she requires intubation due to her poor mental status. Over the course of the next week, her physical exam evolves only minimally, with development of triple flexion in the right lower extremity but no other significant changes. She remains dependent on the ventilator but is otherwise stable. The next step in her medical care is to determine whether to proceed with continued aggressive medical therapy, including tracheostomy and surgical feeding tube (trach and PEG).

C. Siegel
UCLA Department of Neurology, Los Angeles, CA, USA

J. Besbris (✉)
Department of Neurology, Department of Supportive Care Medicine,
Cedars-Sinai Medical Center, Los Angeles, CA, USA

© Springer Nature Switzerland AG 2020
K. Aberger, D. Wang (eds.), *Palliative Skills for Frontline Clinicians*,
https://doi.org/10.1007/978-3-030-44414-3_9

Usual Approach

You approach the patient's family during morning rounds regarding this decision. You inform the family that in order to maintain life, a tracheostomy and PEG tube will need to be placed. Without these, the patient will not be able to eat or protect her airway and will die. You ask the family to please discuss among themselves and then inform the medical team of their decision tomorrow. The family is unsure about what the patient would have wanted in this situation because she never explicitly told them or wrote it down. Some lean toward intervention; others less so but are uncertain and afraid she will die. They finally consent to trach and PEG placement. The procedures are performed, and the patient is shortly thereafter discharged to a long-term acute care (LTAC) facility. There, she is weaned off the ventilator, but does not recover significant strength or language function. She develops multiple decubitus ulcers due to her immobility. She is hospitalized 2 months later for pneumonia, and again 2 months after that for urosepsis.

Palliative Approach

You arrange a meeting with members of the patient's family in a quiet and private space outside of the patient's room. You plan to ask the family to tell you about the patient and her values and to consider what type of life would be acceptable to her. You intend to explicitly state that while there is uncertainty in her prognosis, you can help to provide a range of possible outcomes using current prognostic models, as well as your clinical experience. In order to prepare for the meeting, you review existing data on stroke prognosis and develop a framework of "best case, worse case, and most likely" scenarios in order to give a clear clinical picture of what to expect. You will try to guide family in determining whether trach and PEG will assist the patient in achieving her minimal acceptable outcome. You will also engage in shared decision-making by reflecting on the likely clinical outcomes and how these stack up with the patient's personal values. You will avoid medical jargon and set aside extra time to address any questions that the family has.

Box 9.1 Prognostication in Stroke Is as Equally Necessary as It Is Difficult
Studies of doctor–patient communication have shown that most patients and families appreciate acknowledgement of prognostic uncertainty and want to discuss prognosis even when it is not certain (Evans et al.; Krawczyk et al).

Prognostic indicators may provide some assistance with prediction; however, these tools were not designed to estimate prognosis for individual patients and should not be relied upon as sole predictors of patient outcome. Consideration of individual patient factors and expert clinician assessment remain critically important in developing a prognostic estimate tailored to a particular patient. Below are some commonly used prognostic indicators for stroke, as well as a summary of the outcome that each model would predict for our patient.

Prognostic Indicators for Ischemic Stroke

Prognostic model	Factors included in assessment

I-Score	Age
	NIHSS
	Premorbid cancer or renal disease
	Stroke risk factors:
	    Atrial fibrillation, CHF, previous MI, current smoker
	    Preadmission disability
	    Glucose on arrival

SPAN-100	Age NIHSS
ASTRAL	Age NIHSS Presence of visual field defect Presence of impaired consciousness Time from symptom onset to presentation Glucose on arrival
THRIVE	Age NIHSS History of DM, HTN, atrial fibrillation

You predict using the above prognostic models:

- I-Score: 72.4% likelihood of death at 30 days, 95.8% chance of death or disability at 30 days, 79.6% risk of death or institutionalization at 30 days, and 79.6% likelihood of death at 1 year.
- SPAN-100: Positive (age + NIHSS ≥100) and also was not a candidate for tPA. In a study of 624 patients, 92% of those who were SPAN-100 positive and did not receive tPA had a modified Rankin Scale score of ≥4 at 12 months.
- ASTRAL: >97.1% chance of "poor outcome" at 90 days, defined as a modified Rankin Scale score of 3–6.
- THRIVE: 2% chance of "good outcome" at 90 days, defined as a modified Rankin Scale score of 0–2.

Case Continued – Family Meeting

You meet with the patient's daughter and son. You ask them what they understand about their mother's condition. Her children state that, while they understand she has had a large stroke, they do feel that she is improving as now she has some movement in her right leg. They are anxious to understand how much recovery she might have.

You share that the stroke is affecting a large portion of their mother's brain and has damaged the parts that help her to understand and use language, as well as the parts that control movement and sensation of the right side of her body. You also state that given her age, the size of her stroke, and her other medical problems, you expect her to have lifelong neurological deficits. You validate the family's observation that her leg moves when pinched, but explain that these movements are a type of reflex rather than intentional movement by the patient and are not a sign of improvement.

Box 9.2 Seeing Reflexes Often Given Families Significant Hope

Patients with severe neurological insults may demonstrate nonpurposeful or reflexive movements that may be noticeable to families and can give a false sense of progress or neurological recovery. It is important to both explain to families the significance (or lack thereof) of these movements and also ensure that other team members (e.g., bedside nurse, respiratory therapist) deliver a consistent message in their updates. Additionally, it is important to validate families' hopeful observations because these movements may be very meaningful to them. Even if the movements are not clinically significant, for families this new development can feel like a tremendous leap forward.

You then ask the family about their mother before her stroke. The family states that she was fiercely independent and took pride in her appearance and her tidy home. She loved reading and gardening with her grandchildren. You ask the family to identify the patient's "minimal acceptable outcome," or phrased in common terms, what quality of life would be considered even worse than death. You ask them to reflect on what aspects of her life have been most important to her, and whether there are certain functions or abilities that are so important to her that she would not want to live without them. The family shares that because she took such joy in storytelling and interacting with her grandchildren, she would likely not want to be put through invasive medical procedures if they would not increase the likelihood of being able to communicate with her loved ones. They additionally state that given how deeply she has valued her independence and having her own home, she would not value a life in which she had to live in a facility and rely on staff for her personal care. She had, in fact, made her children promise never to "put her in a nursing home."

You share that it is impossible to predict exactly how much neurologic recovery the patient might have. Although the patient's prognosis is uncertain, you can present statistical data from other patients with similar strokes and cite your clinical experience to guide your best estimate of what might happen. You explain to the family that in the best-case scenario, you expect their mother may regain some strength on the right side and eventually be able to transfer out of bed or walk with assistance. She may also regain a limited amount of language function but will not communicate normally. In the worst-case scenario, the patient may not recover significant function beyond her current state, and you are concerned she may die imminently due to infections or other complications as a consequence of being in the hospital and on a ventilator. The most likely scenario would involve life-long care in a facility, with continued significant weakness and aphasia limiting her ability to walk, talk, or take care of herself.

Box 9.3 Best Case, Worst Case

Discussing prognostic uncertainty can be challenging when a multitude of clinical outcomes are possible. One suggested approach is to outline the "best case, worst case, and most likely" scenarios to help describe the range of potential recovery in a way that is easy to conceptualize, and then compare these scenarios to the patient's minimal acceptable outcome. This allows the provider to help family reflect on whether a patient would want to continue with aggressive treatment for a chance to achieve the most likely clinical outcome or for a smaller chance at the best-anticipated outcome.

You explain that, unfortunately, you do not expect the patient to achieve her minimal acceptable outcome of meaningful communication and independent living. You share that understanding their loved one's goals has helped guide you in your approach to her medical care, and thank the family for their insights. You now recommend stopping aggressive medical treatments, because these are unlikely to result in an acceptable quality of life for the patient. Instead, you recommend palliative extubation and treatment of any symptoms that may be causing her discomfort, rather than potentially prolonging suffering. The family agrees that this feels like the best choice for their loved one.

Box 9.4 Patient-Centered Recommendations
In this case, based on the patient's known values and expected clinical outcome, you are able to make a recommendation to pursue comfort-focused care. This approach to shared decision-making helps to alleviate some of the burden families feel when acting as surrogates for their loved ones. It should be noted that this same approach might have led to an entirely different recommendation if the patient's minimal acceptable outcome matched more closely with the expected clinical outcome. In such a case, recommending trach and PEG placement may have been an appropriate next step. The purpose of shared decision-making is not to limit aggressive medical care in all cases, but to ensure that the type of care a patient receives is concordant with their goals and treatment preferences.

You then also explain that in order to provide rest for her body and allow a natural death without CPR, breathing machines, or other resuscitative procedures, you will now focus on treating symptoms to maximize comfort. The family thanks you for your care and understanding.

Box 9.5 Present Code Status as a Recommendation, Not a Separate Decision
Once a decision is made to transition to a comfort-oriented approach, it is not necessary to discuss code status as "another decision" the family has to make. In this setting, a decision not to intubate or perform CPR is implicit in a transition to comfort-focused care and can be presented to family as part of what this type of care will mean for the patient.

The family is invited to ask any questions they have about the next steps in their mother's care. Her son expresses concern that his mom has not eaten in several days and he worries she will starve. "Wouldn't she be more comfortable if they used a nasogastric tube to feed her?" he asks. You explain that while some patients with severe stroke can enjoy being carefully fed by their families, you do not recommend placing a tube to provide feedings as this is an invasive and uncomfortable intervention that can prolong the patient in her current state. The feeding tube may also increase symptoms such as excess secretions or respiratory distress at the end of life. The family may carefully hand-feed their mother if she shows any signs of hunger, but you add, patients who are actively dying often do not have a desire for food.

Case Conclusion – Palliative Extubation and Transition to Comfort-Focused Care

The family chooses a date for the palliative extubation that allows out-of-town family members to arrive and spend time with their loved one. You explain that most patients die within 24 hours after palliative extubation but that some patients may live several days longer. You assure the family that your team will continue to attentively care for her for as long as she survives. You share that you will give medications, specifically opioids and benzodiazepines, prior to removing the breathing tube so that she does not experience anxiety, shortness of breath, or pain. If she appears to be experiencing any symptoms after extubation, medications will be administered and increased as appropriate. You clarify that these medications are never given with the intention of hastening death. The family is invited to meet with a chaplain, and they request that a priest come before their mother is extubated. After his visit, the family notifies the team that they are ready to proceed. The patient's daughter chooses to stay in the room, while her son opts to wait in the waiting room with the patient's grandchildren. All monitors are turned off to avoid unnecessary alarms during the extubation process, so that the team and family can focus on the patient.

Box 9.6 Palliative Extubation Is Best Treated Like Any Other Medical Procedure

Advance preparation is essential. This includes informing family of what to expect during and after the procedure, making a plan for how to prevent symptoms and having medications available if symptoms do arise, and performing a brief "time-out" before extubation to ensure that all critical staff and family members are present, that all alarms have been turned off, and that any necessary premedications have been given. It is helpful to coordinate with nursing to have extra medication doses readily available and respiratory therapy for their impression on anticipated work of breathing following extubation. If the patient is alert and felt to be at high risk of experiencing respiratory distress, proceed with intermediary step-wise weaning and medication titration instead of abrupt discontinuation. Taking these steps to mitigate the probability post-extubation distress will ease family's memories of this final event.

The patient is extubated and initially appears comfortable, requiring infrequent PRNs for dyspnea. Her need for opioid medications gradually increases as she develops tachypnea and slightly increased work of breathing. She also exhibits periods of agitation, as evidenced by fidgeting in her left arm and associated tachycardia, well managed with haloperidol and lorazepam. She dies comfortably 2 days after extubation, with family at her bedside.

Take-Away Points
1. Patients with devastating stroke may survive for years if provided with aggressive medical care; however, the extent of meaningful neurological recovery may be limited. It is therefore critical to establish the quality of life that is acceptable to the patient before proceeding with aggressive medical care to ensure that the most likely clinical outcome would be acceptable to the patient and to minimize the risk of maintaining a patient in a state that he or she would find unacceptable.
2. Patients and families generally appreciate acknowledgment of prognostic uncertainty during discussions of goals and treatment preferences, and benefit from making shared decisions with the medical team. When prognosis is uncertain, it may be helpful to present a range of outcomes in a "best case, worst case, and most likely scenario" format.
3. Prognostic models may assist with framing possible outcomes and likelihoods for neurologic recovery after a severe stroke, but prognostication should always be tailored to the individual patient.
4. Symptoms of discomfort may be less obvious in patients with neurologic injury resulting in paralysis and/or aphasia. Attention should be paid to subtle signs of discomfort in order to provide adequate symptom management.

References

1. Krawczyk M, Gallagher R. Communicating prognostic uncertainty in potential end-of-life contexts: experiences of family members. BMC Palliative Care. 2016;15:59.
2. Holloway, et al. Palliative and end-of-life Care in Stroke. A statement for healthcare professionals from the AHA/ASA. Stroke. 2014;45:1887–916.
3. Holloway, et al. Estimating and communicating prognosis in advanced neurologic disease. Neurology. 2013;80:764–70.
4. Evans LR. Surrogate decision-makers' perspectives on discussing prognosis in the face of uncertainty. Am J Respir Crit Care Med. 2009;179(1):48–53.
5. Reid JM, Gubitz GJ, Dai D, Reidy Y, Christian C, Counsell C, Dennis M, Phillips SJ. External validation of a six simple variable model of stroke outcome and verification in hyper-acute stroke. J Neurol Neurosurg Psychiatry. 2007;78(12):1390–1.
6. Saposnik, et al. Stroke prognostication using age and NIH stroke scale: SPAN-100. Neurology. 2013;80(1):21–8.
7. Saposnik, et al. IScore: a risk score to predict early death after hospitalization for an acute ischemic stroke. Circulation. 2011;123(7):739–49.
8. Ntaios G, Faouzi M, Ferrari J, Lang W, Vemmos K, Michel P. An integer-based score to predict functional outcome in acute ischemic stroke: the ASTRAL score. Neurology. 2012;78(24):1916–22.

9. Flint AC, Cullen SP, Faigeles BS, Rao VA. Predicting long-term outcome after endovascular stroke treatment: the totaled health risks in vascular events score. AJNR Am J Neuroradiol. 2011;31(7):1192–6.
10. Cooray C, Mazya M, Bottai M, Dorado L, Skoda O, Toni D, Ford GA, Wahlgren N, Ahmed N. External validation of the ASTRAL and DRAGON scores for prediction of functional outcome in stroke. Stroke. 2016;47:1493–9.
11. Flint AC, Kamel H, Rao VA, Cullen SP, Faigeles BS, Smith WS. Validation of the totaled health risks in vascular events (THRIVE) score for outcome prediction in endovascular stroke treatment. Int J Stroke. 2014;9(1):32–9.

Chapter 10
Prognostication and Goals of Care in Advanced Parkinson's Disease

Kevin McGehrin and Christina L. Vaughan

Case Introduction

A 75-year-old man with a nine-year history of Parkinson's disease (PD) with dementia presents to the emergency department with cough, reduced oral intake, and increased agitation. He lives at home with his wife, who is his primary caregiver. Per his wife, he has exhibited significant functional decline over the past year. He previously used a walker, but now relies on a wheelchair. Over the past 6 months, he lost 20 pounds and required two hospitalizations for aspiration pneumonia. His outpatient neurologist simplified his medications due to worsening hallucinations and cognitive impairment. He currently takes carbidopa/levodopa six times a day. Three days ago, he developed a productive cough. Since then, he has become combative and agitated when his wife tries to offer him medications or food that he often refuses. His wife reports that he is now less active and mostly stays in bed. On physical examination, he is afebrile and normotensive. He is inattentive, unable to follow commands, and possibly having visual hallucinations, as he appears to be reaching for invisible items. Neurological examination is notable for hypomimia, diffuse rigidity, and a pill-rolling rest tremor of the left hand. Chest X-ray reveals a right lower lobe infiltrate suggestive of aspiration pneumonia, and he is started on antibiotics. He fails a swallow evaluation, and the speech therapist recommends that he not receive any food or

K. McGehrin (✉)
Department of Neurosciences, University of California – San Diego, San Diego, CA, USA
e-mail: kmcgehrin@health.ucsd.edu

C. L. Vaughan
Department of Neurology, Section of Neuro-Palliative Care, University of Colorado, Anschutz Medical Campus, Aurora, CO, USA

Department of Medicine, Palliative Care Inpatient Consult Service, University of Colorado Hospital, Aurora, CO, USA

© Springer Nature Switzerland AG 2020
K. Aberger, D. Wang (eds.), *Palliative Skills for Frontline Clinicians*,
https://doi.org/10.1007/978-3-030-44414-3_10

medications by mouth. His wife agrees to temporary nasogastric (NG) tube placement for administration of artificial nutrition and medications.

Usual Approach

Neurology is consulted, and you advise that the home regimen of carbidopa/levodopa be continued. For treatment of agitation, the recommendation is quetiapine as needed. You suggest that the patient follow up with his outpatient neurologist after discharge for further medication management. The patient has a prolonged hospital course with poorly controlled agitation, which limits his ability to participate in speech and swallow assessments. After 1 week, he is able to pass a swallow study. He is placed on a modified diet and the NG tube is removed. His wife states that she feels overwhelmed caring for him at home, so he is discharged to a skilled nursing facility. Two weeks later, he returns to the hospital with fever, agitation, and medication non-adherence.

Palliative Approach

Neurology is consulted, but you first perform a comprehensive symptom assessment. You ask the patient's wife to complete the Edmonton Symptom Assessment Scale-Revised: Parkinson's Disease (ESAS-R: PD) [1]. This modified version adds confusion, constipation, stiffness, and dysphagia to the traditional ESAS scale, given the prevalence of these symptoms in patients with PD. [1]

While reviewing the ESAS-R: PD results, you learn that the patient's rigidity has significantly worsened over the past 3 days. This is likely due to missed doses of carbidopa/levodopa. You advise that the patient's home dose of carbidopa/levodopa be continued while he is in the hospital. You also recommend that because meals high in protein can interfere with levodopa absorption, his NG tube feeds should be administered as boluses instead of as a continuous infusion. The tube feeds can be then held for 1 hour before, and after, levodopa administration, allowing for adequate absorption.

> **Box 10.1 Bolus Feed Timing Improves Levodopa Absorption**
> Coordinate bolus feeds to occur 1 hour prior to and after levodopa administration so as to not impair absorption.

You further assess this patient's confusion. The patient's wife mentions that for the past year, he has intermittently seen figures of people in his peripheral vision, particularly at night. These visual hallucinations are not distressing to him. He is normally pleasant, cooperative, and compliant with taking medications; however, for the past 3 days, he has been agitated and argumentative. He frequently accuses his wife of trying to get rid of him or of planning to put him in a nursing home. He yells, "No, no, no!" when offered food or medications and appears to be experiencing visual hallucinations. His agitation is worse at night. His wife recalls similar behaviors when hospitalized with infections in the past. You review his most recent electrocardiogram, which shows a normal QTc interval. You suggest scheduling quetiapine nightly along with as-needed doses available every 6 hours for agitation.

Box 10.2 Quetiapine is Preferred in Parkinson's Disease
Avoid dopamine antagonists (e.g., haloperidol, metoclopramide), which can exacerbate motor symptoms in PD.

While evaluating the ESAS-R: PD results, you learn that this patient has also been constipated with no bowel movements in the past week. The patient's wife reports that normally he has one bowel movement every other day. You recommend starting senokot nightly as initial treatment for the constipation.

In addition to symptom management, you recognize that there are several issues that necessitate a family meeting to discuss this patient's prognosis and plan of care: [2] (Table 10.1):

You prepare for the family meeting by reviewing the literature regarding prognostication in PD and learn that the 50% survival rate is approximately 15 years after diagnosis [3], but the range is quite broad depending on age of diagnosis. Earlier age of onset is associated with longer survival [2]. According to the Centers

Table 10.1 Potential triggers for palliative conversations in Parkinson's disease	
	Accelerated decline in *functional status*
	Behavioral issues including hallucinations, delusions, or wandering
	Bothersome or disabling *pain*, unresponsive to PD medication adjustment
	Caregiver distress or burnout
	Cognitive impairment or dementia
	Existential distress: loss of hope, feelings of despair
	Loss of ability to drive or perform activities of daily living without assistance
	Recent or repeated *hospitalizations* (infections, falls, fractures)
	Significant *dysphagia*
	Weight loss
	Adapted from the Springer textbook Neuropalliative Care – A Guide to Improving the Lives of Patients and Families Affected by Neurologic Disease (2018) [2]

Table 10.2 Risk factors associated with increased mortality in Parkinson's disease

Advancing age [9–11]
Advanced age at onset [8, 9]
BMI < 18 [12]
Dementia [9–11, 13]
Infection [5–8]
Male sex [9, 14]
Psychosis [9]
Reduction in dopaminergic medications due to side effects [12]
Weight loss early in the course [15]

for Disease Control and Prevention, PD is the 14th leading cause of death in the United States [4]. Common causes of death attributed to PD include aspiration pneumonia and falls resulting in serious injuries [5–8]. You review risk factors associated with increased mortality in PD (Table 10.2):

Given the presence of multiple risk factors associated with increased mortality in PD, you realize that this patient is likely nearing the end of his life and is an appropriate candidate for hospice. You learn that patients with PD are less likely to die at home or receive hospice care [16]. Reduced hospice utilization may be due to the high variability of disease progression and the lack of training in palliative care among neurologists [17]. You anticipate that the family meeting will include delivering bad news, specifically that this patient is likely nearing the final months of life. You review the "SPIKES protocol" [18] for delivering bad news to help provide a framework for their upcoming discussion.

Box 10.3 SPIKES Protocol Contains Six Steps to Effectively and Compassionately Disclose Unfavorable Information

The SPIKES acronym consists of *SETTING* up the interview; assessing the patient's (or family's) *PERCEPTION* of their current condition; obtaining the patient's (or family's) *INVITATION* to deliver medical information; giving *KNOWLEDGE* and information to the patient/family; addressing the resultant *EMOTIONS* with empathetic responses; and providing a *STRATEGY* and SUMMARY [18]. In general, the protocol is performed in sequential order, but steps can be revisited based on the flow of the discussion and needs of the patient/family. By approaching this challenging conversation in a stepwise fashion, you hope to exchange information, and then develop a plan that is aligned with the patient's values and goals.

Setting

You schedule a one-hour meeting with the patient's wife in a private conference room. The patient continues to be confused and is unable to participate. Prior to meeting, you ensure that the conference room has adequate chairs and tissues readily available. You silence your cell phone and ask a colleague to respond to pages while the meeting takes place. To start the meeting, you make introductions and thank the patient's wife for taking the time to meet. You ask the wife if there are any other family members or friends who should be included in the discussion. The patient's wife states that she would prefer to have this meeting one-on-one and that she can discuss things afterwards with their other family members. You explain that the goal is to discuss her husband's plan of care and ask if there are any issues that she would like to address today. The wife states that she worries about her husband and would like to discuss plans for what happens once he leaves the hospital.

Perception

You ask the patient's wife to share her understanding of her husband's illness. The wife states that he was healthy his whole life until 9 years ago when he first developed a subtle tremor in his left hand. At that time, she also noticed him walking differently: he appeared "stiff" and "looked depressed" despite saying his mood was fine. His movements seemed slower. Later that year, he lost his balance and fractured his right shoulder. He was evaluated by a neurologist for his gait instability and diagnosed with Parkinson's disease. He was prescribed carbidopa/levodopa, which significantly helped with his bradykinesia and rigidity. He participated in physical therapy for gait training. He functioned independently up until 2 years ago, when he started having more falls. It became difficult to manage his symptoms as he would experience periods of freezing gait, troublesome dyskinesia, and periods when it seemed his medications were not working at all. It seemed as if his neurologist was constantly changing his medications. There was discussion of deep brain stimulation surgery to help with his tremor and motor fluctuations, but her husband did not want to undergo any invasive procedures. Over the past year, his memory has declined significantly. At baseline, he is oriented to self and location but not date. He often forgets recent events and his wife now manages all of their finances, cooking, and medications. When not sleeping, he sits on the couch watching television for most of the day. He suffered several falls this past year resulting in emergency room visits. Because of his falls, he now relies on a wheelchair. In the last 6 months, he has needed to be hospitalized twice for pneumonia and each time he seemed to be "in worse shape afterwards," and never quite fully back to baseline. He frequently becomes agitated and combative, making it challenging for his wife to care for him. She states that she is "exhausted" and not sure how much longer she can continue caring for him at home. She feels guilty about this because in the past he always said that he hated going to the hospital and would never want to be in a nursing facility.

You thank his wife for everything she shared. You ask if she has spoken to their outpatient neurologist about his prognosis and what to expect as his PD progresses. She knows he is declining more quickly now but is unsure how much time he has left. Their outpatient neurologist told her, "Many patients with Parkinson's live long lives, but every patient is different." She assumes her husband will continue to decline and eventually be bedbound, but does not know when that will happen.

You then state, "I want to take a step back and talk about your husband as a person. How would you describe him outside of his Parkinson's disease? What was he like before he got sick? What brings him joy?" The patient's wife sadly says that her husband was always a kind and generous man. He previously had served in the Navy and retired at age 65. She describes his active lifestyle, playing football in his early years, and running marathons as an adult. He loved to travel and read books about American history. The past few years have been hard for him, as he can no longer do many physical activities and is confined to a chair. He does not read because of his poor concentration and memory, but enjoys watching television shows on military history and politics. When asked to name some things that her husband values, she says he appreciates independence and being at home with her. They have been married 40 years. They have no children, but one dog (Rosie). They bought their home the year they married and he has made many renovations since then. He is very proud of that and told her that when he dies, he wants to be at home. When asked to name her husband's fears, she states that he is afraid of being kept alive on machines and in the hospital. When he gets confused at night, it is particularly scary for him to be in an unfamiliar environment. She hopes for him to live peacefully with the time that he has left, and for them to both be happy. She hopes for "more time as his wife, and less time as his caregiver." You thank her for sharing this information. Understanding who he is and what is important to him will help you when making medical recommendations.

Invitation

You ask the patient's wife if it would okay to discuss the details of her husband's medical condition with her and if so, how she prefers to receive medical information. The patient's wife says that she would like to hear any updates regarding her husband's condition and that she prefers to receive medical information directly, with "all the details."

Knowledge

You tell the patient's wife that she has a good understanding of his medical history. You express concern about her husband's decline over the past year, especially with the multiple hospitalizations, and explain that when patients with PD are approaching the end of their lives, they often develop more trouble swallowing, frequent infections, and significant weight loss. You then say, "Unfortunately, I have bad news for you," and after a brief pause, add, "Your husband is dying."

Emotion

You pause again, providing time for the patient's wife to process this information. She appears upset and gazes down at the ground. A minute later you say, "I can see that this must be very difficult for you... I wish I had better news." She agrees that this information is sad to hear, but thanks you for telling her.

Knowledge (Revisited)

The patient's wife then asks "How much time does he have left?" She states that she would like to know this for planning purposes, so that family and friends living out of state are able to see him before he dies. You then explain that physicians can never be completely certain of prognosis, but based on the assessment, her husband likely has weeks-to-months left in his life. The patient's wife appears surprised by this information, but thanks you for being candid with her.

Summary and Strategy

Based on the patient's values and goals, you recommend home hospice services, as this would deliver medical care at home; no more hospitalizations; and continuing support for his wife. You describe the goals of hospice care and answer her questions. Afterwards, you ask the patient's wife to summarize her understanding of the information discussed during their meeting. The patient's wife states she now knows her husband is dying and that transitioning to home hospice services with a focus on comfort is most appropriate, and in line with his goals. You develop a plan with her to place a hospice referral so that she can learn more about available hospice services. You suggest that they meet again the following day to reassess his symptoms and discuss updates regarding his plan of care. The patient's wife agrees.

Case Conclusion

The patient receives one dose of as-needed quetiapine in the morning for agitation with good effect. You up-titrate his scheduled quetiapine regimen to twice daily dosing. The patient has a bowel movement after receiving senokot the night prior. His cognition improves slightly, and he is now able to follow some simple commands and speak in short phrases. Speech therapy reevaluates him and recommends a pureed diet. His NG tube is removed. You meet with the patient and his wife. She mentions that she has spoken with a hospice agency and enrolled him in home hospice services. You and his wife explain the plan of care to her husband, at a level that is appropriate for his cognition. She plans to get additional support at home by hiring caregivers. After hospice services are in place, the patient is discharged home later that day.

Take-Away Points
1. A palliative approach to patients with Parkinson's disease involves both disease-specific symptom management and goals-of-care discussions when appropriate.
2. Prognostication is challenging in Parkinson's disease, but risk factors predictive of increased mortality include recurrent infections, weight loss, dementia, and psychosis.
3. Inpatient management of patients with Parkinson's disease requires special considerations:

   - Constipation is very common and needs prompt identification and management.
   - The timing of levodopa administration is critical. Levodopa should not be administered with meals high in protein as this interferes with its absorption. Tube feeds should be given in boluses (instead of continuous) to allow for adequate levodopa absorption.
   - Dopamine antagonists (e.g., haloperidol, metoclopramide) must be avoided as these medications can exacerbate motor symptoms in Parkinson's disease.

4. The SPIKES protocol is a helpful tool to provide a framework for the delivery of unfavorable news to patients and their families.

References

1. Miyasaki JM, Long J, Mancini D, Moro E, Fox SH, Lang AE, et al. Palliative care for advanced Parkinson disease: an interdisciplinary clinic and new scale, the ESAS-PD. Parkinsonism Relat Disord. 2012;18(Suppl 3):S6–9.
2. Creutzfeldt CJ, Kluger BM, Holloway RG, editors. Neuropalliative care: a guide to improving the lives of patients and families affected by neurologic disease. Cham: Springer International Publishing; 2018. Print
3. Chillag-Talmor O, Giladi N, Linn S, Gurevich T, El-Ad B, Silverman B, et al. Estimation of Parkinson's disease survival in Israeli men and women, using health maintenance organization pharmacy data in a unique approach. J Neurol. 2013;260(1):62–70.
4. Kochanek KD, Murphy SL, Xu J, Tejada-Vera B. Deaths: Final Data for 2014. National Vital Statistics Report. 2016; 65(4). Hyattsville: National Center for Health Statistics.
5. Mappilakkandy R, Pieris A, Miodrag D, Chunduri A. Death in patients with Parkinson's disease – an observational study. Mov Disord. 2017;32(suppl 2):1–8.
6. Su CM, Kung CT, Chen FC, Cheng HH, Hsiao SY, Lai YR, et al. Manifestations and outcomes of patients with parkinson's disease and serious infection in the emergency department. BioMed Res Int. 2018;2018:6014896. https://doi.org/10.1155/2018/601486.
7. Pennington S, Snell K, Lee M, Walker R. The cause of death in idiopathic Parkinson's disease. Parkinsonism Relat Disord. 2010;16(7):434–7.
8. Hely M, Morris J, Traficante R, Reid W, O'Sullivan D, Williamson P. The Sydney multicentre study of Parkinson's disease: progression and mortality at 10 years. J Neurol Neurosurg Psychiatry. 1999;67(3):300–7.
9. Forsaa EB, Larsen JP, Wentzel-Larsen T, Alves G. What predicts mortality in Parkinson disease?: a prospective population-based long-term study. Neurology. 2010;75(14):1270–6.
10. Hughes TA, Ross HF, Mindham RH, Spokes EG. Mortality in Parkinson's disease and its association with dementia and depression. Acta Neurol Scand. 2004;110(2):118–23.
11. Macleod AD, Taylor KS, Counsell CE. Mortality in Parkinson's disease: a systematic review and meta-analysis. Mov Disord. 2014;29(13):1615–22.
12. Goy ER, Bohlig A, Carter J, Ganzini L. Identifying predictors of hospice eligibility in patients with Parkinson disease. Am J Hosp Palliat Care. 2015;32(1):29–33.
13. Louis ED, Marder K, Cote L, Tang M, Mayeux R. Mortality from Parkinson disease. Arch Neurol. 1997;54(3):260–4.
14. Diem-Zangerl A, Seppi K, Wenning GK, Trinka E, Ransmayr G, Oberaigner W, Poewe W. Mortality in Parkinson's disease: a 20-year follow-up study. Mov Disord. 2009;24(6):819–25.
15. Cumming K, Macleod AD, Myint PK, Counsell CE. Early weight loss in parkinsonism predicts poor outcomes: evidence from an incident cohort study. Neurology. 2017;89(22):2254–61.
16. Miyasaki JM, Kluger B. Palliative care for Parkinson's disease: has the time come? Curr Neurol Neurosci Rep. 2015;15(5):26.
17. Robinson M, editor. Case studies in neuropalliative care. Cambridge: Cambridge University Press; 2018. Print
18. Baile WF, Buckman R, Lenzi R, Glober G, Beale EA, Kudekla AP. SPIKES – A six-step protocol for delivering bad news: application to the patient with cancer. Oncologist. 2000;5(4):302–11.

Chapter 11
Saying Yes to Aggressive Measures: The Role of Neuropalliative Care in Critically Ill Patients with Potential for Recovery

Joel Phillips, Brandon Francis, and Justin Voorhees

Case Introduction

Maya is a 20-year-old female who was admitted to an inpatient psychiatric facility for new onset symptoms of irritability, hyper religiosity, repetitive behaviors, and intermittent response to internal stimuli. Prior to this, she was otherwise healthy, gainfully employed, and living independently. Shortly following admission, she develops seizures. CT head and lab studies are unremarkable. A lumbar puncture is obtained and demonstrates anti-N-methyl-D-aspartate receptor (NMDAR) antibodies in the cerebrospinal fluid (CSF). Her seizures do not respond to antiepileptic medications such as lorazepam, valproic acid, and levetiracetam. She is then placed on mechanical ventilation to initiate burst-suppression as the next step to stop her status epilepticus.

NMDAR encephalitis is an autoimmune disorder caused by antibodies that target NMDA neuronal receptors. The classic clinical case of anti-NMDAR encephalitis is young female who presents with new psychotic symptoms such as delusions, hallucinations, agitation, or catatonia. Over the next week, patients develop abnormal movements, seizures, dysautonomia, and alterations in consciousness. These seizures often progress to refractory status epilepticus. The source of NMDAR antibodies is not always found, but almost 60% of young females with NMDAR

J. Phillips (✉)
Hauenstein Neurosciences, Mercy Health Saint Mary's Hospital, Michigan State University, Grand Rapids, MI, USA
e-mail: Joel.Phillips@mercyhealth.com

B. Francis
Department of Neurology and Ophthalmology, Stroke and Neurocritical Care Services, Michigan State University, East Lansing, MI, USA
e-mail: franc221@msu.edu

J. Voorhees
Hospice of Lenawee, Advian, MI, USA
e-mail: jvoorhees@hospiceoflenawee.org

© Springer Nature Switzerland AG 2020
K. Aberger, D. Wang (eds.), *Palliative Skills for Frontline Clinicians*,
https://doi.org/10.1007/978-3-030-44414-3_11

encephalitis will have a teratoma (rare in males). The diagnosis is made through detection of CSF anti-NMDAR antibodies. In a recent literature review, anti-NMDAR encephalitis represented 1% of all intensive care unit admissions for young adults, with median age of 21 years and female predominance (4:1) [1, 2].

Usual Approach

Maya is placed into an induced coma. She is managed with strong sedatives and anti-epileptics. She is evaluated for a teratoma. Her family is told certain procedures and tests will be necessary including tracheostomy, and PEG. Oophorectomy would be introduced with the argument that "this is necessary to save her life." Code status and comfort care are not addressed given her young age. Over her four-month hospitalization, family feels overwhelmed by all the information given to them and are not sure how to process it. They meet an encyclopedia of consultants; sometimes clinicians do not seem up to speed or on the same page. Because they are not sure what to hope for, therefore they constantly feel disappointed. They experience a whirlwind of emotions, and this experience creates rifts in several of their inter-family relationships.

Palliative Approach

As Maya's neurocritical care specialist, you recognize the importance of early palliative care involvement given prognostic uncertainty and family's need for support. You invite the palliative team into Maya's care shortly after intubation. Palliative care builds significant rapport with the family. They describe the long course ahead and explore with the family how Maya's path may look, based on treatment options, her values and character, and definitions of quality of life. They share that Maya is an ambitious career woman, a socialite, and never one to pass up an adventure. With

> **Box 11.1 Early Palliative Care Involvement Amplifies and Does Not Limit Care**
> Building rapport with families and ascertaining patient values helps decision-making remain patient-focused. Early palliative care involvement, especially for emotionally charged cases such as with young patients, helps facilitate this groundwork from the beginning of the treatment course. Palliative care is recommended for all critically ill patients irrespective of prognosis [3, 4]. Currently, palliative care is often consulted late in the illness course to discuss hospice or comfort care, creating a perception that they only intervene at the very end of life [5]. When this happens, this becomes a self-fulfilling prophecy. Moreover, the patients, families, and clinical teams then miss out on the valuable benefit of continual support throughout this distressing process of critical illness.

the palliative team jointly, you ensure a consistent message in gently laying out best and worst cases of her condition, and the real possibility of a poor prognosis given her prolonged status epilepticus. Through shared decision-making, the family decides to continue burst suppression, the standard for curative care, because she would always "seize any opportunity" available to her.

You initiate Maya on midazolam, phenobarbital, and ketamine infusions. In a series of meetings in tandem with the palliative team, you meet with the core family members to discuss riskier management and diagnostics. With their agreement, you initiate rituximab in hopes of decreasing antibody production. You evaluate for neoplastic etiologies with imaging. CT, MRI, and ultrasounds are unremarkable. A PET scan suggests hepatic flair with a possible colonic lesion. Colonoscopy is introduced and accepted, although unfortunately is unremarkable. Trials of lifting burst suppression are not tolerated; she remains in status epilepticus. After 2 weeks, despite these interventions and workup, you have no positive news to share. Nevertheless, throughout this process Maya's family feels well prepared and respected and appreciates your team for taking the time to sit with them daily in this uncertainty.

The next clinical consideration now is tracheostomy and PEG. The clinical teams

Box 11.2 Does the Absence of Good News Equate to Bad News?
As clinicians, we must remember that caring for patients (and families) is grounded in caring for them, not defined by clinical outcomes. "Good news" is not always possible. However, it is still valuable to make time to sit with them even if we are uncomfortable with our clinical progress, hear their concerns and stories, and honor their perspectives.

are feeling distress about this young woman. You hear one of the clinicians express discouragement about her prospect of recovery, and that comfort care might be best. Another bristles at this remark, pointing out her young age and that she "deserves a chance." You recognize that you yourself also feel some discomfort discussing a non-full care option with the family of this young patient; after all, you are a parent yourself and this hits close to home.

Box 11.3 Counter-Transference Is Unavoidable
Nearly all clinicians can identify a certain type of patient phenotype (e.g., demographic, illness, behavior) that is difficult for them. Patients may consciously or subconsciously remind them of their child of similar age, a recent close loss, a strained dynamic with a family member of their own. Maintaining objectivity is simply not always possible. Despite our best attempts at complete rationality, we bring our values, our experiences, and our lives into interactions with the people we care for daily. Importantly, we should not fault ourselves for being human and nor should we expect that these emotional experiences do not influence our care.

You invite the broader family to a goals-of-care meeting with your team and the palliative team. Although you have seen several of these people before at various points in the day, this is the first time you have addressed them altogether. You invite them to share their reflections on Maya. They tell more stories about her: celebrating her recent promotion at work, her steady boyfriend who has already been adopted into the family, her thrill-seeking hobbies, and her uncanny persistence in always speaking her mind.

Pivoting the mood, her older brother asks, "So what happens now?" With their collective permission for your honesty, you provide a succinct, simple summary: "Despite our best care, we have not seen Maya improve, nor have we arrived any closer to understanding why this is happening to her." Pausing to gather yourself, you explore next steps, achieving a delicate balance between their hope for cure and a new treatment course option. You gently introduce the idea of focusing exclusively on comfort instead, including compassionate extubation, aggressive symptom management, and allowing natural death without resuscitation. At this, Maya's younger sister bursts into tears, "I can't see her like this anymore. This isn't her. She's dying!" Multiple family members begin heated exchanges with one another. You allow several minutes for everybody to speak their mind, facilitating discussion by inviting quiet members to chime in if they would like. With a pause in the conversation, you interject by asking, "If the healthy Maya could be in this room right now, and see herself in this state, what would she say to all of you?" The tone shifts, and everybody is in agreement that Maya would wish to continue full care. Maya's mother, who has felt torn seeing her children disagree while wrestling with her own feelings, states as you finish the meeting, "Thank you for reminding us to keep Maya's wishes at the center. How she has always lived her life points us to knowing the path she would choose for herself."

Box 11.4 Whose Decision Is It Anyway?

Just as it is difficult for clinicians to completely and always separate their feelings from their care, families and surrogate decision-makers also differentiate what they think the patient themselves would want with what they would want for them. The fear of losing their loved one may cause the latter to obscure the former. One helpful question to clarify the difference is, "What are you most worried about right now?" Realizing that the patient's own wishes exist outside of their own feelings may relieve them of feeling impossibly burdened by a difficult decision.

Maya undergoes a tracheostomy and PEG tube placement. She continues burst suppression and standard–of-care treatment with immunotherapy including steroids, plasmapheresis, intravenous immunoglobulin, cyclophosphamide, and bortesamib [6–8]. Despite a negative pelvic ultrasound, statistically an ovarian micro-teratoma is still the most likely etiology [9, 10], in which case resection would eliminate antibody production and usually lead to seizure control.

Gynecologic oncology is consulted for bilateral oophorectomy, and join you and the palliative team for a difficult, emotional family meeting. The implications on future family planning and infertility are weighed against a potentially lifesaving surgical intervention. Scenarios with positive and negative ovarian pathology results are thoughtfully explored with the family. They understand surgery may not alleviate her condition; however, in line with the prior meeting they believe Maya would wish to proceed.

Box 11.5 It Takes a Village
Over the course of weeks, this patient's care spanned multiple specialists, and within each specialist multiple clinicians given rotating inpatient schedules. The palliative team remained the constant presence and "held the patient and family's story," helping coordinate and communicate across care teams and onboard new faces. Through this extra layer of support, they maintained the family's trust that all of her clinical teams were working together to give Maya the best care possible.

Case Conclusion

After surgery, the pathology report returns negative for neoplasm. Her family was adequately prepared. They mourn the loss of Maya's future fertility; however, they remain steadfast in the hope that she will still recover. Over the next 6 weeks, her seizure activity surprisingly diminishes on her current treatment regimen, and she is subsequently weaned off anti-elliptic medications. She slowly begins to communicate and regain function. Your team and the palliative team help the family gradually share news of her hospital course with Maya, including the oopherectomy. She is ultimately transitioned to a long-term care facility. After her 4-month hospitalization and six months of rehabilitation, Maya is now driving, dating, and back to work.

Box 11.6 Palliative Care Is Imperative for Families in Neurocritical Illness
Longitudinal palliative support is imperative for families in neurocritical illness. Neurologic injury is often sudden, with a prolonged recovery. Families are suddenly placed in surrogate decision-maker roles and experience emotional distress which may later result in anxiety, depression, and posttraumatic distress disorder, referred to as postintensive care syndrome-family (PICS-F) [11, 12]. Palliative should be involved regardless of timing or prognosis [13] and improve family satisfaction with communication and trust [12].

Take-Away Points

1. Early palliative care involvement amplifies and does not limit neurocritical care management by establishing groundwork for patient-centered decision-making and supporting families through prognostic uncertainty.
2. Even when there are no favorable clinical updates, the continuum of care and rapport can be maintained by making time to sit with families, hearing their concerns and stories, and honoring their perspectives.
3. Counter-transference is experienced by all clinicians and influences the delivery of care. Awareness, not suppression, is the ideal approach.
4. Surrogate decision-makers may conflate their feelings for the patient with their understanding of what the patient would want for themselves. Asking "What are you most worried about right now?" may help clarify this misattribution and ease the decision process.
5. Palliative care is imperative for families in neurocritical illness, improves satisfaction with communication and trust, and reduces postintensive care syndrome.

References

1. Kayser MS, Dalmau J. Anti-NMDA Receptor Encephalitis in Psychiatry. CPSR. 2011;7:189–93.
2. Dalmau J, Graus F. Antibody-Mediated Encephalitis. N Engl J Med. 2018;378:840–51. https://doi.org/10.1056/NEJMra1708712.
3. Munro C, Savel R. Aggressive care and palliative care. Am J Crit Care. 2018;27:84–6. https://doi.org/10.4037/ajcc2018757.
4. Harmon S. Psychiatric and palliative care in the intensive care unit. Crit Care Clin. 2017;33:735–43. https://doi.org/10.1016/j.ccc.2017.03.010.
5. Tabibian B, et al. Transitioning the treatment paradigm: how early palliative care service involvement affects the end-of-life course for critically ill patients in the neuro-intensive care unit. J Palliat Med. 2018;21. [Epub ahead of print].
6. Scheibe F, et al. Bortezomib for treatment of therapy-refractory anti-NMDA receptor encephalitis. Neurology. 2017;88:366–70. https://doi.org/10.1212/WNL.0000000000003536.
7. Titulaer M, et al. Treatment and prognostic factors for long-term outcome in patients with anti-NMDA receptor encephalitis: an observational cohort study. Lancet Neurol. 2013;12:157–65. https://doi.org/10.1016/S1474-4422(12)70310-1.
8. Lwanga A, et al. Occult teratoma in a case of N-methyl-D-aspartate receptor encephalitis. Neuroradiol J. 2018;31:415–9. https://doi.org/10.1177/1971400918763578.
9. TANYI JL, MARSH EB, Dalmau J, CHU CS. Reversible paraneoplastic encephalitis in three patients with ovarian neoplasms. Acta Obstet Gynecol Scand. 2012;91:630–4. https://doi.org/10.1111/j.1600-0412.2011.01365.x.
10. Boeck A-L, et al. Ovarectomy despite negative imaging in anti-NMDA receptor encephalitis: effective even late. Case Reports in Neurol Med. 2013;2013:1–3. https://doi.org/10.1155/2013/843192.
11. Knies A, Hwang D. Palliative care practice in neurocritical care. Semin Neurol. 2016;36:631–41. https://doi.org/10.1055/s-0036-1592358.

12. Davidson J, et al. Guidelines for family-centered care in the neonatal, pediatric, and adult intensive care unit. Crit Care Med. 2017;45:103–28. https://doi.org/10.1097/CCM.0000000000002169.
13. Frontera J, et al. Integrating palliative care into the care of neurocritically ill patients: a report from the improving palliative care in the ICU project advisory board and the center to advance palliative care. Crit Care Med. 2015;43:1964–77. https://doi.org/10.1097/CCM.0000000000001131.

Chapter 12
"I am a Fighter": Recognizing and Responding to Cancer Metaphors

Rushil Patel and Andrew Epstein

Case Introduction

Ms. W is a 65-year-old woman with Stage IIA ER+/PR+/HER2- breast cancer initially diagnosed and treated 7 years ago. One year ago, she was found to have metastases in the pelvis, femur, vertebra, and liver. She was treated with letrozole and radiation, but her cancer progressed. She has been hospitalized several times for cord compression (treated non-operatively), worsening ascites secondary to acute kidney injury (AKI) and liver dysfunction, and deep venous thrombosis (DVT). Now 1 week after her more recent hospitalization, she is admitted for uncontrolled pain, hypotension, and a 3-point drop in her hemoglobin. The ED physician asks about her code status, and she is labeled as a full code. Her wishes are again confirmed by the admitting ICU team. She definitively tells them, "I want everything done. I am a fighter." Her family nods their heads defiantly.

Usual Approach

Ms. W is transferred to the ICU and receives the full scope of interventions: CT abdomen/pelvis to investigate bleeding; central line placement; pressor support; and a plan for CPR and mechanical ventilation should she code. No source of bleeding

R. Patel (✉)
Supportive Care Service, Memorial Sloan Kettering Cancer Center, New York, NY, USA

A. Epstein
Supportive Care Service, Memorial Sloan Kettering Cancer Center, New York, NY, USA

Gastrointestinal Oncology Service, Memorial Sloan Kettering Cancer Center, New York, NY, USA

Department of Medicine, Weill Cornell Medical College, New York, NY, USA

© Springer Nature Switzerland AG 2020
K. Aberger, D. Wang (eds.), *Palliative Skills for Frontline Clinicians*,
https://doi.org/10.1007/978-3-030-44414-3_12

is identified. Gastroenterology is consulted, but an esophagogastroduodenoscopy (EGD) is deferred given hemodynamic instability and poor prognosis. She continues to decline and is intubated. Clinical teams, including oncology, repeatedly suggest, "Withdraw care," to her family. They do not agree based on her stated wishes. Eventually, the patient dies after a prolonged code in the ICU.

Palliative Approach

As the consulting oncologist, your partners have cared for Ms. W and her family for many years; however, you are new to them. Your review of her clinical details clearly indicates that she is at the end-stage of her cancer and escalating ICU interventions would likely only prolong her decline. You introduce yourself to Ms. W, her sister at bedside (her health care proxy), and other family members. You observe that Ms. W appears profoundly more cachectic and debilitated since, as described in her last office visit. You gently share your concern that although her clinical teams will attempt to identify treatable issues (e.g., bleeding), you are worried that nothing reversible may be found. You ask Ms. W what she has ever thought about should her condition worsen further. She states, "Resuscitation." You ask her to clarify, and she explains, "Don't stop. I'm a fighter."

> **Box 12.1 "Fighting" Does Not Always Mean the Same Thing**
> Violence metaphors should not be interpreted as a desire for more intervention but rather an invitation to explore associated values and emotions.

You pause to consider this charged word: "fighter." You hear various kinds of metaphors from your patients and families as they have made meaning of their experience of illness. At times, you yourself have used them, consciously and subconsciously, in discussions with them. After all, metaphors allow one to articulate an abstract concept in a relatable way [1]. You consider common metaphor frameworks:

Violence metaphors in cancer – is it really about fighting?

Violence metaphors permeate oncology, as they often do in other contexts, such as the "war on drugs," the "war on poverty," and even the "war on Alzheimer's" [1]. In cancer care, these metaphors become entrenched: physicians as commanders, patients as combatants, and the care team as allies [2].

These metaphors, though widespread, belie the patient experience. Cancer invades from within, so an individual wages war with oneself. Cancer-directed treatments are "weapons"; however, they not only affect cancer cells but can also result in significant morbidity, which is atypical of warfare. And regardless of the "victor," patients experience psychological, spiritual, and social stressors as they proceed in this journey. Playing the role of co-conspirators, patients may hesitate to disclose these kinds of distress for concern of upsetting their caregivers and their physicians [3].

Ultimately, wars require winners and losers. Survivors may be winners but calling them so diminishes their need for extended healing. Survivors are left with anxiety, perception of increased risk, and greater likelihood of depression; the need for extended healing is diminished [4]. The losers, or those for whom the cancer no longer responds to treatment, perceive their predicament as a personal failure: "Patients fail treatment instead of treatment failing patients." [2, 5] This charged language undermines the role of palliative care, especially when cancer-directed therapy is exhausted, and the focus shifts to quality of life [2, 6, 7].

Journey metaphors in cancer – focused on the present and not the outcome

Apart from violence metaphors, journey metaphors are also prevalent in patient stories of their experiences with illness and treatment and present cancer as a shared experience [8]. Advocates for this metaphor cite the need to dissociate the absence of recovery from a result of personal failure [9, 10] and to engage emotions associated with connection [8].

Empowerment vs disempowerment – how metaphors define the patient experience

One way to approach violent or journey metaphors used by patients and families is to identify whether they signify either *empowerment* or *disempowerment* in the face of their illness [10]. In one study of online writings of health professionals and patients, empowering violence metaphors reflected purpose, pride, and camaraderie, while empowering journey metaphors reflected camaraderie and control. Disempowering metaphors for both subtypes reflected vulnerability and passivity [10].

Empowerment Metaphors

Metaphor	Subtype	Examples
Patient successfully fighting the disease	Violence	"I am such a fighter." "[I am] ready to kick some cancer butt."
Patient successfully fighting health professionals	Violence	A patient describes a successful outcome in a consultation as "winning that battle." After expressing dissatisfaction with her wound care, another patient comments that now she has "another thing to beat my surgeon up about."

Metaphor	Subtype	Examples
Mutual encouragement and solidarity	Violence	Some patients praise others for being "fighters" and for "winning the battle" against cancer. "Soldier on everybody."
Patient as a traveler in charge of the journey	Journey	Conveys control and acknowledges positive moments: "My journey may not be smooth but it certainly makes me look up and take notice of the scenery!" Another patient points out that, even after I have "gone as far as I can, I can push myself that little bit further.'"
Patients as travelling companions	Journey	"Rocks in our paths are easier to handle when we're all in it together." "The best people to help you are the ones who've been there before or are heading there with you."

Adapted from [10]

Disempowerment Metaphors

Metaphor	Subtype	Examples
Disease fighting the patient	Violence	A patient describes her breast cancer as a "killer" that "strangles and shocks your soul." A particularly strong sense of vulnerability is expressed as "time bombs" while in remission.
Patient unsuccessfully fighting the disease	Violence	"I feel such a failure that I am not winning this battle."
Treatment fighting the patient	Violence	Chemotherapy is described as giving the patient's body "a hammering" or "a battering."
Patient as a traveler on a difficult journey	Journey	One patient comments that the journey is "like trying to drive a coach and horses uphill with no back wheels on the coach.'"
Patient travelling without control over their journey	Journey	One patient talks about a "reluctant journey," while another wonders how she can "navigate this road" that she does "not even want to be on."

Adapted from [10]

Case Continued – Palliative Approach

From Ms. W's language choice, you clearly sense that she is empowered by her violence metaphor. You first align with her empowerment before helping her reframe her goals by asking, "What are you fighting for?" She replies, "To get stronger to be at home with my daughter." You encourage her to continue thinking about these questions as her teams continue their diagnostics.

Over the next few days, Ms. W receives several transfusions with normalization of her blood counts. An IVC filter is placed. She does not require pressors or ventilatory support and is transferred to the floor within 48 hours in stable condition.

The following day, you ask her, "In our first meeting, you identified yourself as a fighter, and we discussed what you were fighting for. I was wondering if we could spend some time exploring how this fight has affected you." She replies, "I feel weak and have no energy to do the things I enjoy, like caring for my daughter. She has bipolar disorder and really struggles sometimes to maintain a job and take care of herself. I usually spend most of my day with her." You recognize that this is not only her reason for fighting but likely also where she finds her identity and purpose.

Box 12.2 "Fighting" Should Always Beget More Questions About the "Fight"

Hearing the word *fighting* should trigger a knee-jerk reflex, an invitation to follow-up. Two helpful questions to ask are:

- "What are you fighting for?" may provide a glimpse into priorities and short/long-term goals.
- "How has this fight affected you?" redirects the patient away from the future best-case scenario to instead consider tangible milestones and concerns in the present.

You speak with her outpatient palliative care physician who has been co-following along with your oncology colleagues over the last year. Since he started seeing Ms. W at time of diagnosis of her incurable metastatic disease, he has cultivated a deep relationship with her and her family. Sensing similar needs as you have observed, he has met with Ms. W and her family separately. In a private conversation, Ms. W's sister shared with him that the patient had told her she could not imagine living without the ability to communicate and help her daughter.

Over the next few days, Ms. W continues to decline. Additional family, including her sisters, have now arrived in town. You host another family meeting and facilitate small group discussion, inviting each of them to share their concerns and hopes. Everyone agrees that their hope is for the patient to make it home, although they fully understand she has worsened precipitously. You look at her sisters and ask, "What would it be for Ms. W's daughter to lose her mom?" The sisters look hesitantly at the patient, who nods and express that they will support their niece no matter what happens to Ms. W. They give Ms. W permission to focus on herself, to be less selfless in her own needs. A weight seems to lift from Ms. W's shoulders. She says to you, "I don't like talking about this kind of future, but it does give me some peace." You consider making another recommendation to exclusively focus on comfort; however, you realize that pushing Ms. W to make a decision that is incongruent with her identity would only tarnish the significant healing that has already occurred today for her family (Table 12.1).

The next day, the patient develops refractory hypotension. She responds minimally to temporizing measures including IV fluids, pressors, and steroids. She no longer retains decisional capacity. You approach her sisters and family and recommend allowing a natural death. They feel you have guided and prepared them well for this moment and agree with exclusive focus on comfort. They appreciate that you allowed Ms. W to go through this final process on her own terms and using her own words. They deeply respect that you highlighted and honored her greatest priority, which was to know her daughter would be protected. Ms. W dies comfortable with her family and daughter at bedside.

Table 12.1 Exploratory responses to common metaphors

Patient's Responses	Pitfall	Recommended Responses	Rationale
"I'm a fighter."	Providers assume individuals prioritize cancer-directed treatments above all else and miss the opportunity to explore goals and values [6, 11].	"What motivates you in this effort? "What are you fighting for?" "How has this fight affected you?	Explore goals and values to better align treatment plan.
"I survived cancer." "I beat cancer."	The word "survivor" invokes war and diminishes recognition of need for extended healing and recovery following treatment. Patients are left with more anxiety, perception of increased risk, and greater likelihood of depression [4].	"I sense how important the success of the treatment has been. What are you now able to do that you couldn't before?" "How you are handling the adjustment back to your regular responsibilities?"	Redirects focus to recovery and identifies post-treatment needs.
"Without treatment, I feel like I'm giving up."	Cancer progression is perceived as a personal failure versus the limits of cancer-directed therapy.	"What are you hoping to gain by treating the cancer?" "What worries you most right now?"	Explore goals and values to better align treatment plan.

Take-Away Points
1. Both violence and journey metaphors are frequently used by patients to make meaning of their illness experience.
2. "Fighting" metaphors are opportunities to trigger follow-up questions about what is being fought for and how the fight has been.
3. Metaphors should not be interpreted as answers to questions about interventions but should instead be explored to elicit underlying goals and values.

References

1. George DR, Whitehouse ER, Whitehouse PJ. Asking more of our metaphors: narrative strategies to end the "war on Alzheimer's" and humanize cognitive aging. Am J Bioeth. 2016;16(10):22–4. https://doi.org/10.1080/15265161.2016.1214307.
2. Reisfield GM, Wilson GR. Use of metaphor in the discourse on Cancer. J Clin Oncol. 2004;22(19):4024–7. https://doi.org/10.1200/JCO.2004.03.136.
3. Byrne A, Ellershaw J, Holcombe C, Salmon P. Patients' experience of cancer: evidence of the role of "fighting" in collusive clinical communication. Patient Educ Couns. 2002;48(1):15–21. https://doi.org/10.1016/S0738-3991(02)00094-0.
4. Hoffman KE, McCarthy EP, Recklitis CJ, Ng AK. Psychological distress in long-term survivors of adult-onset Cancer. Arch Intern Med. 2009;169(14):1274. https://doi.org/10.1001/archinternmed.2009.179.
5. Miller RS, et al. Oncol Times. 2010;32(12):20. https://doi.org/10.1097/01.COT.0000383777.50536.b2.
6. Malm H. Military metaphors and their contribution to the problems of overdiagnosis and overtreatment in the "war" against cancer. Am J Bioeth. 2016;16(10):19–21. https://doi.org/10.1080/15265161.2016.1214331.
7. Trachsel M. Killing the pain and battling the lethargy: misleading military metaphors in palliative care. Am J Bioeth. 2016;16(10):24–5. https://doi.org/10.1080/15265161.2016.1214310.
8. Perrault S, O'Keefe MM. Journeys as shared human experiences. Am J Bioeth. 2016;16(10):13–5. https://doi.org/10.1080/15265161.2016.1214319.
9. Harrington KJ. The use of metaphor in discourse about cancer: a review of the literature. Clin J Oncol Nurs. 2012;16(4):408. https://doi.org/10.1188/12.CJON.
10. Semino E, Demjén Z, Demmen J, et al. The online use of violence and journey metaphors by patients with cancer, as compared with health professionals: a mixed methods study. BMJ Support Palliat Care. 2017;7(1):60–6. https://doi.org/10.1136/bmjspcare-2014-000785.
11. Shapiro J. "Violence" in medicine: necessary and unnecessary, intentional and unintentional. Philos Ethics Humanit Med. 2018;13(1):1–8. https://doi.org/10.1186/s13010-018-0059-y.

Chapter 13
"What Does the Awake Ventilated Patient Really Want?": Shared Decision-Making in the ICU

Lauren Goodman

Case Introduction

A 56-year-old man is transferred from a local long-term acute care hospital (LTACH) to the intensive care unit (ICU) at a regional tertiary care academic cancer hospital. He has lung cancer metastatic to brain and was receiving maintenance chemotherapy until 3 months ago. He was hospitalized 5 weeks ago with respiratory failure, failed extubation, and then tracheostomy. He was not tolerating ventilator weaning at the LTACH.

He is awake and alert on the ventilator, and by nodding, mouthing, or writing, signals that he is short of breath and anxious. He is tachycardic, normotensive, and has coarse breaths sounds bilaterally without wheezes or rales. With ventilator settings on assist control, rate 12, tidal volume at ideal body weight, PEEP 6, and FiO$_2$ 30%, he has SpO$_2$ 92% and RR up to 30s.

During this ICU stay, he has failed weaning trials due to increased work of breathing and anxiety despite scheduled and PRN medications for both complaints. Repeat imaging shows progression of metastatic disease in his lungs and brain, and oncology (both the consulting team and his primary oncologist) has evaluated that due to his poor functional status, he is not a candidate for further chemotherapy.

His wife expresses her wish to take him home with a ventilator and continue disease-directed therapies, including physical therapy, in the hope of getting him strong enough to receive further chemotherapy.

L. Goodman (✉)
Department of Internal Medicine, Division of Pulmonary, Critical Care and Sleep, The Ohio State University Wexner Medical Center, Columbus, OH, USA

© Springer Nature Switzerland AG 2020
K. Aberger, D. Wang (eds.), *Palliative Skills for Frontline Clinicians*,
https://doi.org/10.1007/978-3-030-44414-3_13

Usual Approach

Given multiple barriers to communication, the clinical teams turn to the patient's wife to serve as his surrogate decision-maker and guide treatment goals. His input is not solicited. They discuss prognosis and treatment options clearly and succinctly. She appreciates their candor but states that she has heard this before and resolves to continue full medical care, with the hope that he may receive further chemotherapy. She says, "He told me he's not ready to give up yet."

Over the next 2 weeks, he is able to slowly wean off the ventilator. He appears increasingly withdrawn. He returns to the LTACH but is hospitalized again monthly for urinary tract infection, pneumonia, and other complications. Chemotherapy is never reintroduced as an option. A few months later, he develops pressor-refractory shock, PEA arrest. Further resuscitation is unsuccessful.

Palliative Approach

You meet with the patient and his wife and explain that while her perspective has been invaluable, you very much want her husband to be the center of today's conversation.

Because the patient is awake and alert, you evaluate his capacity and allow him to express his values and preferences even if he cannot make decisions.

Box 13.1 Communication with Nonverbal Patients
For patients who retain fine motor abilities, try pen/paper, dry erase boards, or typing on a smart device or laptop. If motor control is impaired, gesturing toward a letter board may be more effective. Speech therapists may have access to specialized boards for patients with locked-in syndrome. Some ventilator-dependent patients may tolerate an in-line speaking valve if the ventilator can provide leak compensation. Some patients with tracheostomies or even endotracheal tubes are able to enunciate with their lips sufficiently to be understood through lip-reading. Some patients with tracheostomies can produce fricative speech, making sounds with sharp movements of their lips and tongue without requiring air movement through their vocal cords.

This patient is unable to tolerate the reduced ventilator support provided with the inline speaking valve but is able to steady his hands to write clearly enough with pen and paper to be understood. He mouths words clearly to communicate simpler responses as well. This process of receiving his thoughts and questions takes much longer than a typical spoken conversation but provides him opportunity to have his questions and concerns answered, express his values and preferences, and direct and control his care as much as possible.

You begin the conversation by assessing for adequate symptom management. Goals-of-care conversations can already be frustrating for patients with communication challenges; poorly controlled pain, dyspnea, nausea, or anxiety significantly limit the discussion quality. He reports that the scheduled anxiolytics you prescribed have helped him, and he thanks you for this thoughtfulness.

Next, you assess for capacity. You start with the orientation question, making sure to avoid the propensity of only asking "yes" answer questions. You then further evaluate his ability to appreciate his current situation. You inquire about how life used to be like before this illness, what he misses most, what he looks forward to these days, and how he imagines his life may be in the future. He expresses that he understands his cancer has progressed and is no longer treatable. He no longer is able to enjoy his prior hobbies, and he cannot accept the image of his present self. He knows that the ventilator is keeping him alive, but just knowing that he is "living this way always connected" brings him severe anxiety.

Now knowing him better, you segue into the decision-making part of the conversation. You begin by asking him how much he wishes to know.

Table 13.2 Do Not Assume All Patients Wish to Know Their Prognosis
While clinicians tend to believe knowledge is power, we must be careful not to impose this worldview onto others. When faced with the prospect of bad news, patients have a right to defer medical updates and decision-making to their surrogates. For some patients, knowledge may bring more distress. It is not an essential component of their decisional process and may involve placing a greater trust in someone else, a spiritual belief, or even blissful ignorance. Always first ask both the patient and all present parties if they would wish to receive your honest information.

The patient appreciates your invitation and earnestly asks you to be frank with him. You provide a medical update using minimal jargon, outlining his failure to improve, progression of cancer, and absence of further cancer-directed treatment. You do discuss that it may be possible for him to leave the ICU and return to a facility. Importantly, you also raise the very real possibility that even with the best medical treatments, he may remain in this state that he already finds unsatisfying. Although this conversation takes a long time, he thanks you for taking the time to share this with him.

After thoughtfully considering this juncture, he expresses that he is tired, and without a reasonable certainty that he would return home in the near future, he does not find it meaningful to continue living this way. He requests some time to say goodbye to his family, and to change the focus of his care in the ICU to comfort exclusively and allow his natural death off of the ventilator "as a whole man again."

His wife is startled as she did not know he felt this way. "This isn't him," she says. He responds, "Well, I know this was what you wanted for me, and the docs didn't really ask before, but a lot has happened since then." She appears anxious and asks for the rest of the day to speak with him in private. You allow them space for these weighty conversations. You ask for the palliative care team to support them as well.

The following day, you meet with them again. You first address the patient, and ask if his intentions have changed since yesterday. He recalls your conversation and expresses the same views. His wife candidly shares, "I'm scared of losing him. But now I know where his heart is, and although I don't agree with him, I love him, and I can't put my own feelings before his."

Box 13.3 Consistency Is Essential to Capacity
While all the elements of capacity are valuable (communicability, under-standing, appreciation, and rationalization), the importance of consistency is often understated. Consistency over time lends powerful support to a deeply rationalized decision. Often following abrupt insults, such as a trau-matic amputation, or waking up in the ICU after an unexpected event, patients may express desire for less care or even passive suicidality. Over time (potentially as short as days), and with engagement with their support network, they may adjust to the sense of a "new normal" baseline and such decisions revert.

Having reached closure, the patient wishes to expedite this process and asks for ventilator discontinuation later today. This is particularly difficult for his wife to accept because it is her birthday. However, with support from the palliative team chaplain, she reframes her thinking from "my birthday will always be the day my husband died' to 'my birthday will always be an important day I share with my husband."

Case Continued

After his family arrives and spends time with him to say goodbye, he indicates to the nursing staff that he is ready to transition off the ventilator.

Usual Approach

He is started on a morphine drip at 1 mg/hr. After 1 hour, his dyspnea remains severe; the nurse reports this to the intern who agrees to double the morphine drip rate. After another hour, dyspnea remains uncontrolled, and the intern and nurse double the drip again to 4 mg/hr. This pattern continues every few hours; the following morning his drip is running at 48 mg/hr, and he is very sleepy but still with intermittent respiratory distress and increasing myoclonus. His family is very upset and exhausted from constantly monitoring his symptoms and asking the nurse to intervene further.

> **Box 13.4 Opioid Infusions Take 4–5 Half-lives to Reach Steady State**
> Starting an opioid infusion at 1 mg/hr will not enable the patient to experience "1 mg per hour" of morphine until at least a half day later. Bolus opioids are more effective for uncontrolled symptoms at any point in the comfort care process. Likewise, changing an opioid infusion will again require the same amount of time before the increased dose takes full effect. Importantly, decreasing the infusion follows the same pharmacokinetic timeline.

Palliative Approach

The plan for transition to comfort care is discussed among the ICU physicians, nurses, aides, chaplain, and respiratory therapists. The area outside his room is kept as quiet and calm as possible. Multiple chairs are brought into the room for family to be able to sit, both at the patient's side and slightly away from the patient when they need to. A tray of beverages and snacks is brought for family so they can stay with the patient without having to leave the room for nourishment. A small family room in the waiting room is designated for family members to gather as needed outside of his room as well. The hospital chaplain offers to visit; the patient and family accept, and she participates in prayers along with the family's pastor who is also visiting.

His wife continues to watch the patient's vital signs on the telemetry monitor, distracted from her husband, until the nurse gently informs her that she will be removing the telemetry leads and pulse oximetry probe and turning off the monitor for the patient's comfort. Initially, his wife is hesitant to allow this, but once the monitor is shut off, his wife is able to focus on her husband, to talk with him, and to share stories with their family.

Once everybody feels ready, the patient is given morphine and lorazepam approximately 20 minutes prior to the ventilator being discontinued to allow the medications to reach peak effect. Then, the respiratory therapist turns off the ventilator and places him on a tracheostomy mask, with his trach cuff deflated as tolerated. He is able to speak a few words intermittently. After this transition, the room becomes quiet and the family more tense as they wait for additional words from him.

The nurse asks the patient if he would like any music playing or the television on. He requests Elvis; she plays an internet radio station in his room, and he smiles and relaxes. Family members smile too as they hear his favorite songs playing and start to tell stories about him that they associate with these songs.

A fan is kept at the bedside to help with his dyspnea, as several studies have shown a fan or medical air are at least as effective as oxygen in treating dyspnea. He is given bolus doses of morphine 15 minutes apart to treat his dyspnea. This interval allows for assessment at peak effect prior to adding further doses, minimizing unnecessary sedation. His mother expresses concern that this will "kill him faster." The palliative and ICU physicians assure her that his symptoms and medication effects are being monitored, and that he is being given medication only as much and as often as his symptoms require. They gently inform her that multiple studies have shown that judicious use of opioids and benzodiazepines do not hasten death. He does not become significantly sleepy with the morphine doses, and he is asked to rate his anxiety and is asked whether he wants lorazepam. At times, he wants the medication and becomes somewhat sleepy with it; at other times, especially shortly after family members arrive, he declines it and remains alert as long as he wishes.

After a few hours off the ventilator, he indicates it is more important to him to keep his anxiety and dyspnea better controlled, even if it means he will be sleepy. He is given scheduled doses of both morphine and lorazepam based on his usage over the preceding hours, and as-needed doses are continued as well. He continues to express that control over his symptoms is insufficient and that he wants to be asleep rather than continue to experience these symptoms. Lorazepam and morphine are now scheduled given his increasing needs and permission for double effect given his stated preference. A few hours later, he has a relaxed face with easy work of breathing. He dies comfortably over the next 12 hours, with family resting at his bedside.

Take-Away Points
1. Any patient with capacity and desire to participate in decision-making must be given the opportunity to do so. Many different methods can be used to facilitate communication with ventilated patients, whether they are orally intubated or have a tracheostomy.
2. Do not assume all patients wish to know medical knowledge/prognosis; always ask before you tell.
3. Appropriately administered symptom management medications do not hasten death.
4. Symptom management is achieved first with intermittent bolus doses of opioids and benzodiazepines rather than starting with infusions (which require five half-lives, i.e., many hours, to reach steady-state full effect).

Chapter 14
A Mother's Love – Support Despite Disagreeing with Goals of Care

Neha Shah

Case Introduction

A 47 year-old woman with pleomorphic cutaneous T-cell lymphoma is admitted for difficulty breathing and lethargy. She has been receiving chemotherapy and radiation at her local academic center. Her last oncology appointment was 2 weeks ago where she was told that her cancer had progressed. She is intubated in the ED for respiratory failure and admitted to the ICU. Subsequently she is diagnosed with tricuspid valve endocarditis and septic shock from MRSA bacteremia. Her mother is her primary caregiver.

Usual Approach

Full ICU sepsis care including IV fluids, antibiotics, and ventilator support with weaning trials. Her respiratory failure and mental status improve, and she is downgraded to the floor and then discharged home with peripherally inserted central line (PICC) access and a prolonged course of antibiotics.

If she does not improve in the first weeks of ICU treatment, a tracheostomy and PEG tube are placed, and she is transferred to an long term acute care hospital (LTACH).

N. Shah (✉)
Piedmont Healthcare, Georgia, GA, USA
e-mail: Neha.Shah@piedmont.org

© Springer Nature Switzerland AG 2020
K. Aberger, D. Wang (eds.), *Palliative Skills for Frontline Clinicians*,
https://doi.org/10.1007/978-3-030-44414-3_14

Palliative Approach

Daily multidisciplinary rounds in the ICU include the intensivist, nurse, physical therapist, respiratory therapist, dietician, pharmacist, case manager, and palliative care team liaison. When you round on this patient during her first week in the ICU, her mother appears tired, haggard, frail, and in emotional distress. You approach her after your rounds and introduce yourself with a hug.

Box 14.1 Therapeutic Touch
More than your knowledge, your patients want to know that you truly care about them and their loved ones. You find that patients/families in distress sometimes really appreciate a hug. You have never been turned down for a hug in 18 years of practicing medicine. It brings the human touch back and conveys, "I am here with you, in this moment." It can also soften bad news without diluting the message.

She clings to you and says she really needed support. She asks if we can meet the next day. The next day, your patient remains ventilated, sedated, and unresponsive. About 10 different drips are running, including pressors, sedatives, and antibiotics. There is a putrid smell emanating from her body. She has extensive skin lesions covering her body from her cancer with bacterial superinfection.

Before you address her mother, you pause to observe the situation in the room. You notice that her mother has gospel music playing. She has put up pictures of her daughter when she was better from 5 years ago. Kleenex from home, not the hospital ones, are on the bedside table. (It is obviously not her first time crying, and she wants good tissues.) She also has a large bag of her clothes in the corner; she is prepared to camp out. She is pacing the room. You offer another hug and ask her to come to a quiet room to talk.

Box 14.2 Assess the Situation, Not Just the Patient
Build a habit of assessing nonverbal cues – appearance of the room, music, faith tradition items, and emotional state of present family. Asking about pictures present, or stored on cell phones, creates a natural connection and provides a sense of the patient's character.

You ask about her daughter's journey. She accepts the invitation and starts talking slowly: Over the pasts 3 years, she has been receiving chemo and radiation that don't seem to have helped, and with numerous concerns with the port/PICC lines and infections. Up until 3 months ago, she was still working full-time. She found significant meaning and identity in her job; she was due for a promotion. Since then, she has had a rapid decline, is now unable to work, and has become depressed. Her

Table 14.1 FICA tool for spiritual assessment

	Questions to ask
*F*aith and belief	Do you have spiritual believes that help you cope with stress?
*I*mportance	What role do your beliefs have in regaining health?
*C*ommunity	Are you part of a religious or spiritual community? If so, is this of support to you and how?
*A*ddress in care	How would you like me as your health care professional to address these issues in care?

Table 14.2 AMEN protocol – honoring spirituality in our patients and surrogates

*A*ffirm the patient's belief. Validate his or her position.	"How wonderful that would be. I am hopeful, too."
*M*eet the patient or family member where they are.	"Tell me more about what you hope the miracle will look like" "I join you in hoping (or praying) for a miracle."
*E*ducate from your role as a medical provider.	"While I recognize I only play one role in this bigger process, would you allow me to share my medical perspective on what's going on?"
*N*o matter what, assure the patient and family you are committed to them.	"No matter what happens, I will be with you every step of the way." "I don't claim to have a crystal ball, but I can commit to being honest and transparent with you on this journey"

mother is her main support; she is single and unattached, and her father died many years ago.

You then ask her mother what her own sources of strength have been as she has partnered with her daughter. She readily talks about her faith. Instead of feeling awkward about the topic, you instinctively recognize how necessary it is to explore these values, as they are central to patient and surrogate decision-making (Table 14.1) [1].

She believes God may have a miracle for her daughter. You gently ask, "What will happen to your daughter after this life?" She is unafraid and answers with confidence, "She's going to Heaven." When you ask what miracle she is praying for, she wishes for her daughter to wake up and speak to her again (Table 14.2) [2].

Box 14.3 Miracles Do Happen

In addition to exploring primary hopes/miracles, it is also valuable to inquire further about smaller hopes. This can help families expand their consideration of different clinical scenarios. They may also identify other needs on how best support them (e.g., family reconciliation, supporting young children).

In complex ICU cases with unclear prognostication, families sometimes share that they have observed miracles but not necessarily the ones they imagined. A CVA patient may not wake up but may open his eyes briefly and "squeeze hands" one last time. A septic patient on five pressors may hold on just long enough for an important family member to finally arrive before dying. While these miracles may seem small, they are nonetheless made meaningful by families and often contribute to closure. Celebrate them.

Her mom appreciates your support but mentions that other clinical staff have repeatedly asked her about code status over the last 24 hours. She feels that everybody is ready to "give up" on her daughter. She is her daughter's "prayer warrior" and knows that her daughter is determined to live. One time she shared with her mother that she wanted her to "fight for me until the end."

Recognizing the frustration of decision-fatigue, you reassure her that no decisions must be made today. You validate her feelings and ask if you could provide anticipatory guidance with best-case/worst-case scenarios.

Because of the rapport you have built, she agrees to hear this. You share: "In the best case, her infection improves and organs recover. She may wake again and breathe on her own, and even leave the hospital to a nursing facility. However, she'll need weeks of antibiotics and likely won't be eligible to resume cancer treatments for a while." She nods her head slowly. You continue: "In the worst case, she isn't able to breathe without the machine, her organs weaken further, and she may never wake up to be herself again. She would receive additional small surgeries to enable her to live on machines in a long-term hospital." Hearing this, her mother shakes her head with conviction. You also introduce an alternative comfort-oriented approach. Hearing this, she says, "I hate that word, comfortable. Pain is part of illness." You affirm both her strength and her daughter's, and rephrase it gently: "If your daughter begins to die, I would like her to not suffer, and instead allow the process to be natural and her body to be at peace." She nods silently.

You summarize with a recommendation: "Let us continue what we are doing for now, and if she is not showing the improvement that we are hoping for, we will come together again and discuss again how to proceed. For now we will continue to pray and hope for that best case." She agrees and trusts your guidance. You ask what she wants to say to her daughter, assuring that she can hear, and she says she wants you to pray with them together.

Box 14.4 Praying with Families

In Judeo-Christian and Catholic traditions, prayer in times of poor health allows people to seek God's comfort, discernment, and intercession. Often they may ask their clinicians to join them in these sacred and vulnerable moments. Some clinicians may share their patient's faith systems, and others may not. You are never obligated to participate if it is unacceptable to your own values; instead offer the assistance of a hospital chaplain if available. If, however, your position is more flexible, consider joining into this therapeutic alliance with patients and their families. Simply bowing your head and holding a respectful moment of silence will suffice.

When you return later in the day, the patient's pastor is visiting. At their request, you pray with them. Afterwards, the pastor asks to speak with you. You review the clinical situation, and he shares he has been here many times before with other families. He offers to be a supportive guide to the patient's mother should the patient worsen. He has seen the patient decline over the last few months and recalls some words she shared with him privately and will spiritually ground her mother when difficult decisions approach. You thank him for his care for them, and he does likewise.

Over the next 3 days, the patient deteriorates. She is now in Acute Respiratory Distress Syndrome (ARDS) with escalating pressor requirements. You meet with the mother again. Building on your last conversation, you describe compassionate wean and extubation. She agrees and believes that giving her daughter a natural death would preserve her dignity; however, she wants this to happen at their home. You recall that some hospice agencies will transfer home on the ventilator and then shortly thereafter perform a controlled compassionate wean and extubation. However, you recognize that this patient is not stable enough to go home. You share with her the bad news. Nonetheless, she is insistent that her daughter remains full code and full care until she can be safely transferred home to die. You share your concern with her that time is likely short.

She holds vigil at the bedside, praying ceaselessly. You hear her say, almost to herself, "I should have never made her come in." You pause and realize that she is so adamant about insisting on a full code because of guilt. You gently ask her to tell you more. "She told me she was dying," she says, "and that she wanted to stay home. I made her come in. Now I have to get her home: She wants to die there." You try to support her but know that this is a deep-seated need for her now. Before you leave for the day, you call her pastor and ask him to support her as well.

As you drive home that night, you think about this mother and daughter and hope that she will make it until the morning. In the evening, you receive a call from the ICU team pleading with you to "help the mother understand." The patient has already coded three times with return of spontaneous circulation (ROSC) achieved each time. On the phone, her mother remains adamant about continuing resuscitation efforts. She tearfully shares: "I know what's going on, and that my baby is in God's hands. He keeps starting her heart again. I need to respect her wishes, I need to fight for her until the end." You validate her needs and support her decisions, and instruct the ICU team to continue. The ICU team calls again hours later to report that the fourth code was unsuccessful, and at time of death, the mother thanked and hugged each of them.

The next day, you and your ICU team debrief about the distress of having to deliver futile care to a dying patient. This is a learning case for everyone involved. Decision made by patients and surrogates and how you are care for them are rooted in much more than knowledge.

Box 14.5 You Do Not Have Just One Patient, but Many
Not every dying patient in the ICU needs a comfort care death. Non- beneficial (previously referred to as futile) care may be frustrating, and clinicians are never obligated to provide it; however, there may be circumstances in which doing so would result in less harm. Your patient's family has become

your patient as well. Although death is a certain outcome for the patient, you may yet have a significant lasting impact on these individuals who will remember this experience forever. As with this patient, sometimes allowing non-beneficial treatment (e.g., continuing to code the patient) may grant the survivors a modicum of peace and closure. Non-maleficence can extend beyond the patient to include their families as well.

Take-Away Points
1. Therapeutic touch and nonverbal cues augment your clinical expertise in care for patients and their families
2. Spirituality is a core component of many patients' and surrogates' decision-making frameworks. The FICA spiritual assessment and AMEN protocol will help you not only better understand your patients but also increase their trust in your ability to care for them in a meaningful way.
3. Miracles often do happen in the ICU, and although they may manifest differently than what was originally requested, they are nonetheless meaningful.
4. If personally acceptable, joining passively in prayer with families when requested may strengthen therapeutic alliances.
5. Non-beneficial care may sometimes nonetheless be beneficial for families, and allowing a reasonable degree of leniency may facilitate closure.

References

1. Rhonda S. Cooper M, Anna Ferguson RN, Joann N. Bodurtha, and Thomas J. Smith. AMEN in Challenging Conversations: Bridging the Gaps Between Faith, Hope, and Medicine. J Oncol Pract. 2014;10(4):e191–e195. https://www.ncbi.nlm.nih.gov/pmc/articles/PMC4870587/.
2. Puchalski C, & Romer AL. Taking a spiritual history allows clinicians to understand patients more fully. Journal of palliative medicine. 2000;3(1):129–37.

Chapter 15
End-Stage Renal Disease and Shared Decision-Making Dilemmas

Indra D. Daniels

Case Introduction

You are the nephrologist who has assumed care of Mr. ST, an 88-year-old man admitted several days ago with shortness of breath and dependent edema. He is being treated for acute-on-chronic heart failure and acute cardiorenal syndrome. Cardiac catheterization 2 months ago showed severe inoperable triple-vessel heart disease and diastolic dysfunction with a preserved left ventricular ejection fraction. His medical history includes stage III chronic kidney disease, hypertension, diabetes mellitus type II, hyperlipidemia, gastrointestinal bleeding, and transient ischemic attack. This is his fourth admission in a year.

Since admission, Mr. ST has remained volume-overloaded, and your associate has advised dialysis. Mr. ST is now receiving a furosemide infusion and is slightly improved. He needed noninvasive positive pressure ventilation (NIPPV) for a few days but is now on supplemental oxygen via nasal cannula. Two months ago, he had similar symptoms, and his creatinine peaked at 4.4 mg/dl but has hovered at about 3.0 mg/dl since then. His vital signs have been stable for the past day, and he is sitting up in bed, able to recount his medical history, and talk about his goals of care.

Usual Approach

You inform Mr. ST the risks of dialysis, such as hypotension during treatment, but assure him that dialysis will help him.

I. D. Daniels (✉)
Nephrology and Hospice & Palliative Medicine, Attending Physician, Palliative Care Service
Mount Sinai South Nassau, Oceanside, NY, USA

Icahn School of Medicine at Mount Sinai, Oceanside, NY, USA

© Springer Nature Switzerland AG 2020
K. Aberger, D. Wang (eds.), *Palliative Skills for Frontline Clinicians*,
https://doi.org/10.1007/978-3-030-44414-3_15

You advise him that he will need temporary venous access for dialysis and that you will contact a surgeon. You tell him that he will also need a permanent access, likely an arteriovenous (AV) fistula or graft in his arm, for long-term dialysis.

Palliative Approach

Key questions to consider:

- *How much does Mr. ST know about his cardiac and renal condition?*
- *How much does he understand about dialysis?*
- *Will dialysis really help him?*
- *What are his goals of care?*

Mr. ST is actually fairly knowledgeable about his illness and says his cardiologist is concerned about him undergoing procedures, as he is at high risk for dying during surgery. Mr. ST says he is not interested in dialysis. He understands that while dialysis may help him feel better, it will not change his underlying disease. He thinks hemodialysis, vascular access creation, and trips to an outpatient unit would be burdensome. His brother had a "good" end-of-life experience and was "comfortable" with home hospice services a year ago, and he wishes for the same.

You leave Mr. ST's room with plans to pursue conservative non-dialytic management of end-stage renal disease (ESRD), in keeping with his goals of care. During the visit, you specifically asked Mr. ST about advance directives. As an attentive nephrologist, you do not regard advance directives within the purview of any "other" specialist or discipline; therefore, you are willing to address the matter with him.

Mr. ST completes a Medical Orders for Life Sustaining Treatment (MOLST) form with you, which includes Do Not Rescuscitate (DNR) and Do Not Intubate (DNI) orders. The cardiologist agrees with you on placing a hospice referral. You assure Mr. ST that you will speak with his granddaughter, Ms. KH, who is his surrogate for health-care decisions, but you are unable to contact her.

Box 15.1 Frailty, Risk Stratification, Prognostic Tools
Nephrologists can employ several approaches to dialysis discussions. A paternalistic approach views initiation of dialysis a success. An informative approach focuses on patients' values and quality of life and presents conservative management as an option. A more interpretive approach takes this a step further and offers treatment recommendations [1].

Chronic kidney disease (CKD) and ESRD patients want to have information on their treatment options, and treatment needs to be focused on the patients' goals and values, not on family or physician preference. Projected mortality statistics can be helpful in goals of care discussions, but quality of life on dialysis cannot be ignored. One study of 200 patients >70 years of age documented significant time lost in hospital admissions, travel, treatment time, and posttreatment fatigue in hemodialysis patients [2]. Peritoneal dialysis, too, can be burdensome for frail elderly patients with impaired physical or cognitive function [3].

The 2010 Renal Physicians Association (RPA) guidelines clearly recommend that patients forgo dialysis if their prognosis is already limited by virtue of age, advanced dementia, severe hypotension, or severe malnutrition, to name but a few comorbidities [4]. Instead of steering patients toward dialysis, consider conservative management of patients in selected patients. A conservative approach does not mean "do not treat." Care will continue to target anemia, volume status, bone disease, cardiovascular risk factors, and electrolyte abnormalities. Concurrent palliative care would address patient goals, identify and treat pain and other symptoms, provide psychosocial and spiritual care, advance care planning, and allow early identification of increasing care needs and hospice eligibility.

Does offering conservative non-dialytic treatment mean giving up on the patient? Several studies have shown no statistically significant survival advantage of dialysis over conservative treatment among patients 80 years or older [5–7]. A recent Austrian study of over 8000 patients showed that the survival benefit of dialysis did not persist beyond 2 months compared to survivors of the conservative group [7].

How do you identify patients who might not benefit from dialysis? Several prognostic scoring systems have arisen in the last few years, especially noting higher mortality risk in elderly ESRD patients [6–10]. Key indicators that suggest poor outcomes with dialysis include impaired functional status with the Karnofsky score less than 40, severe chronic malnutrition with albumin less than 2.5 g/dl, and multiple comorbidities in patients 75 years or older.

While prognostic clarity is valuable for nephrologists, avoid carrying jargon into goals-of-care conversation (e.g., survival percentages, quality-of-life estimates). Instead, integrate recommendations into patient's desired functional goals. If patients agree readily to dialysis, do not concur without reflection. Make sure to explore reasons behind the patient's request. Misconceptions about survival benefit or quality of life are common. Above all, listen to the patient. Ask about their hopes, expectations, and concerns. Determine circumstances under which the patient would consider forgoing or stopping therapy [11, 12].

Two days later, you return to see Mr. ST and discover that in your absence, he has agreed to your associate's recommendation to start dialysis to manage volume overload. He has also agreed to placement of an AV fistula, which you consider risky and unwarranted, considering his multiple comorbidities.

In discussion with the patient, you learn that his own wishes do not match those of his family. While his own feelings about dialysis are unchanged, he feels conflicted because he knows his children want him to accept dialysis. The patient says his family "aren't ready to say goodbye yet" and want him "to keep fighting." Ultimately, he chose to follow whatever his granddaughter wanted for him, as this was more important to him than his own wishes.

Box 15.2 When My Wishes Are Not My Own

Patients reserve the right to defer their decision-making capacity to others at any time. For patients who are intimately connected, they may choose to follow another's wishes instead of their own. Often this occurs when the patient feels that they could cause significant emotional distress to that individual, and this creates a greater aversion than forgoing their own agency. This pattern can be seen between devoted couples, parent–child dyads, and in certain cultural contexts.

Mr. ST undergoes placement of a temporary dialysis catheter and an AV fistula and starts dialysis treatments. Nevertheless, his condition deteriorates, he develops rapid atrial fibrillation, rectal bleeding, pneumonia, and acute respiratory failure. He is hospitalized for an additional 2 weeks, ultimately discharged to a skilled nursing facility, and experiences progressive functional decline during the months leading to his death. His family never accepts a hospice model of care, which would have focused on his comfort, despite Mr. ST articulating his preferences.

Box 15.3 Should an AV fistula Be Placed in this Patient with Advanced Heart Disease and Cardiorenal Syndrome?

Although many guidelines recommend a fistula-first as preferred vascular access, patients with short prognoses warrant a broader palliative consideration [13].

Remember that AV fistulas require at least a month, sometimes 6–9 months before they are suitable for cannulation, and sometimes patients are subjected to further surgery when fistulas fail to mature.

In a palliative setting, the insertion of an AV graft or a tunneled dialysis catheter is more appropriate than a fistula. Some grafts can be used in as little as 24 hours after creation. In general, grafts can be used within approximately 1 week, which is most appropriate for an elderly patient with 1 month to one-year life expectancy. Furthermore, a central venous catheter can be useful, despite risks of infection or thrombosis, if patients only require a very limited treatment course.

Find a balance between patients' expected survival, access survival, and potential complications. Comorbidities such as peripheral vascular disease and heart failure can compromise cardiac output; accesses can thrombose easily if a patient's blood pressure suddenly drops on hemodialysis.

Take-Away Points

1. Use an interpretive approach to goals of care: elicit patients' values, hopes, and concerns, and then distill them into patient-centered recommendations.
2. Think about conservative non-dialytic treatment as an option, particularly in frail patients.
3. Patients may rationally choose to follow a surrogate's desires for their care above their own wishes.
4. AV grafts may be a better vascular access choice than fistulas in patients starting dialyses with limited prognoses.

References

1. Ladin K, et al. Characterizing approaches to dialysis decision-making with older adults: a qualitative study of nephrologists. Clin J Am Soc Nephrol. 2018;13(8):1188–96.
2. Carson R, et al. Is maximum conservative management an equivalent treatment option to dialysis for elderly patients with significant comorbid disease? Clin J Am Soc Nephrol. 2009;4(10):1611–9.
3. Brown EA. Peritoneal or hemodialysis for the frail elderly patient, the choice of 2 evils? Kidney Int. 2017;91(2):294–303.
4. Renal Physicians Association. Shared decision-making in the appropriate initiation and withdrawal from dialysis: clinical practice guideline. 2nd ed. Rockville: Renal Physicians Association; 2010.
5. Verberne W, et al. Comparative survival among older adults with advanced kidney disease managed conservatively versus with dialysis. Clin J Am Soc Nephrol. 2016;11(4):633–40.
6. Thamer M, et al. Predicting early death among elderly dialysis patients: development and validation of a risk score to assist shared decision making for dialysis initiation. Am J Kidney Dis. 2015;66(6):1024–32.
7. Reindl-Schwaighofer R, et al. Survival analysis of conservative vs. dialysis treatment of elderly patients with CKD stage 5. PLoS One. 2017;12(7):e0181345.
8. Beddhu S, et al. A simple comorbidity scale predicts clinical outcomes and costs in dialysis patients. Am J Med. 2000;108(8):609–13.
9. Couchoud CG, et al. Development of a risk stratification algorithm to improve patient-centered care and decision making for incident elderly patients with end-stage renal disease. Kidney Int. 2015;88:1178–86.
10. Cohen LM, et al. Predicting six-month mortality for patients who are on maintenance hemodialysis. Clin J Am Soc Nephrol. 2010;5(1):72–9.
11. Davison SN, et al. Executive summary of the KDIGO controversies conference on supportive care in chronic kidney disease: developing a roadmap to improving quality care. Kidney Int. 2015;88(3):447–59.
12. Rak A, et al. Palliative care for patients with end-stage renal disease: approach to treatment that aims to improve quality of life and relieve suffering for patients (and families) with chronic illnesses. Clin Kidney J. 2017 Feb;10(1):68–73.
13. Woo K, Lok CE. New insights into dialysis vascular access: what is the optimal vascular access type and timing of access creation in CKD and dialysis patients? Clin J Am Soc Nephrol. 2016 Aug 8;11(8):1487–94.

Chapter 16
Discontinuing Continuous Renal Replacement Therapy in the Intensive Care Unit

Tamara Rubenzik

Case Introduction

Your patient, AO, is an 86-year-old male with end-stage renal disease (ESRD) on intermittent hemodialysis, congestive heart failure (ejection fraction 35%), and aortic stenosis who underwent transcatheter aortic valve replacement (TAVR) one year ago who was admitted to the ICU five days ago with shortness of breath, volume overload, and hypotension. He is being managed with slow volume removal via continuous renal replacement therapy (CRRT), and simultaneously requiring two pressors due to hypotension and concern for cardiogenic shock. He is awake, alert, and able to engage in conversation with you during your visits. Today, he reports mild shortness of breath, but no other complaints. You note, however, that he has not had any improvement in his clinical condition despite five days in the ICU, and the ICU team has been unable to find a definitive cause for his persistent hypotension.

AO has been on dialysis for eight years and had been doing reasonably well until his aortic stenosis became so severe last year that he required an aortic valve replacement. At that time, he was not deemed to be a good candidate for a surgical aortic valve replacement and thus underwent a TAVR. Since this procedure, he has had a slow decline in his functional status, and this is currently his third admission in 2 months for cardiac-related issues. AO's brother, who has been at his bedside daily, turns to you and asks, "Doc, is he getting any better?"

T. Rubenzik (✉)
Departments of Nephrology and Palliative Care, University of California San Diego, San Diego, CA, USA

© Springer Nature Switzerland AG 2020
K. Aberger, D. Wang (eds.), *Palliative Skills for Frontline Clinicians*, https://doi.org/10.1007/978-3-030-44414-3_16

Usual Approach

At this point, the usual response might be one of encouragement. You reply by saying, "Well, his breathing is improving and that is a good sign. We just need to give the ICU a bit more time to help your brother." AO continues on CRRT in the ICU for days to weeks without any change in his mental status, but develops slowly worsening hypotension leading to escalation of vasopressor support eventually preventing further fluid removal. His brother receives regular *updates* from the nephrology and ICU teams about small daily progress or setbacks, but no mention is made of the global picture that AO continues to decline despite prolonged ICU care. He agrees to intubation one day to "help his lungs" and is shocked to hear for the first time a few days later that his brother may die in the hospital.

Palliative Approach

Following his last admission, you had planned to speak with AO about his code status and goals of care, though you were not sure how he might handle the topic, given he had come out of the hospital only one month ago. Unfortunately, he was hospitalized again before you had the chance to try.

> **Box 16.1 Kidney Disease Patients Desire Goals-of-Care Conversations**
> The literature shows that patients with advanced chronic kidney disease (CKD) and ESRD want to discuss prognosis, goals of care, and end-of-life care with their medical providers. A large survey of advanced CKD and ESRD patient showed that while the majority are comfortable discussing end-of-life issues with their family and medical teams, very few are having conversations about prognosis and end-of-life preferences with their nephrologists [1]. Other studies evaluating nephrology fellows and practicing nephrologists have found that, despite patient preferences toward having conversations about end-of-life decisions, most providers do not feel prepared for these difficult conversations [2, 3].

You know that AO is not doing well. Given his numerous comorbidities, especially ESRD, he is at increased risk of dying in the hospital.

> **Box 16.2 ESRD can be a Worse Prognostic Indicator Than Cancer**
> Male patients with ESRD who are 75 years of age or older have an adjusted mortality four times greater than age-matched Medicare beneficiaries and more than 2.5 times greater than age-matched Medicare beneficiaries with cancer. Dialysis patients are less likely to use hospice and more likely to die in the hospital than age- and comorbidity-matched Medicare beneficiaries [4, 5]

In an attempt to ease into conversation with the patient and his brother about AO's poor prognosis, you use hope and worry statements to gently share bad news. You tell him that you hope he will get better, but he has not improved since his arrival to the ICU and you are worried that he might not survive this hospitalization. AO seems to be listening, but does not respond verbally or with any change in his facial expressions. His brother does not seem completely surprised to hear this, but you can see that he needs some time to process this information.

Hope/Worry Statements

Hope/worry statements allow you to align yourself with patients and families, demonstrating that you not only hear them but are invested in their emotions. They simultaneously provide an opportunity to introduce and test pivots into bad news. Ensure a noticeable pause before transitioning into the worry component of the statement.

"I hope that his breathing will get better…	… and I worry that he may never leave the hospital"
"I hope that the infection can be treated…	…and I worry that the damage already done to his organs is beyond repair."
"I hope he will wake up again…	…and I worry that he will never again be the man you remember him to be."
"I hope that his spirit will continue to be so strong…	…and I worry that his body is showing that it is getting tired."

AO's brother asks to meet again after allowing the patient additional time. You agree and also clarify milestones for what improvement would look like. "Right now he is on numerous forms of life support – oxygen for breathing, medications to boost his blood pressure, and kidney replacement." You share that hope would be to be on less support when you reconvene.

Over the next three days, the patient's clinical condition has failed to improve. He continues to require supplemental oxygen. You have not been able to wean his pressor requirement to maintain slow CRRT volume removal. He has completed antibiotics without noted benefit. You meet again with AO, his brother, and also his sister at bedside for a goals-of-care conversation, and use the PERSON mnemonic as a guide [6].

PERSON Framework for Goals of Care

This helps you navigate the discussion as you obtain patient and family understanding of his current illness, explore who the patient was before he became ill, and use this information to determine the best course of action for current and future medical care.

*P*erception: Patient and family understanding of current health status
*E*xplore: Explore who the patient was before his illness
*R*elate: Relate the prior level of functioning to current health status, give a medical update, and use both to guide decisions
*S*ources of worry: Inquire about new worries following the discussion
*O*utline: Outline the current plan
*N*otify: Inform other care providers of the plan

You begin the conversation asking if it is permissible to speak frankly to all parties present, especially since you have not met his sister before. AO does not wish to participate but rather listen, and answers that he trusts his brother fully to make decisions for him. His siblings tell you that they do not understand what is wrong with him currently, but they have seen him slowly deteriorate since he underwent his TAVR. He has been spending more time in the hospital than at home over the last two months, and his sister, a retired nurse, is worried that he is coming to the end of his life. She is tearful, stating she doesn't want her brother to suffer. You discuss that AO used to be an active man, living independently, cooking his own food, and maintaining a garden. Since his TAVR, however, he has moved in with his brother and has been unable to care for himself. Over the last two months, he has indeed spent more time in the hospital than at home.

They ask you if he is going to improve. You distill all his current medical complexity into the context of what you have just learned. "It sounds like AO's quality of life has been steadily worsening since the TAVR one year ago, and he has already lost many of the joys in his life. I think this hospitalization is now a tipping point, where despite being on several forms of life support he has not gotten better. I worry that he won't be able to leave the hospital, and that he may be slowly dying." You leave sufficient time for this weighty statement to sink in. AO turns to his brother and says simply, "This isn't life for me. I am not scared." AO's sister asks what can be done to prevent unnecessary suffering for her brother. They agree to a transition to comfort care, including stopping pressors in addition to CRRT, and focusing intently on keeping him comfortable.

You give the patient and his family some time to spend together and leave to update the ICU team. Though they agree with his poor prognosis, the intensivist is shocked to hear that a decision has been made to stop CRRT. They cite the patient's alertness and normal mental status as a reason to continue renal replacement therapy.

Box 16.4 Managing Colleague Distress

Doctors and other healthcare team members (e.g., nurses, respiratory therapists) may show significant distress with a decision for comfort care when the patient is not imminently dying or if there is a perception that we can "do more." This is especially difficult when the patient is lucid and/or young. They may be considering their own personal/family experiences, faith traditions, or value systems. Acknowledging colleagues' distress as normal, and addressing their emotions can assist them in accepting these difficult situations. If helpful, keep patient and family autonomy at the center of such reflections, allowing there to be many "right views" but only one "best view" for this case.

You acknowledge the difficulty and emotion involved with this case. You have a detailed discussion with the ICU team about the patient and/or caregiver's ability to choose to forego dialysis as outlined in the Renal Physician Association's Clinical Practice Guideline on Shared Decision Making in the Appropriate Initiation of and Withdrawal from Dialysis.

Renal Guidelines for Starting, Stopping, and Withholding Dialysis

The RPA guidelines review ten key steps for choosing to start, stop, or withhold dialysis for patients with advanced CKD, acute kidney injury (AKI), and ESRD. Relevant to this case, it is appropriate to withdraw dialysis in a patient who has decision-making capacity and has requested it be discontinued [7]

Recommendation No. 1: Develop a physician–patient relationship for shared decision-making.

Recommendation No. 2: Fully inform AKI, stage 4 and 5 CKD, and ESRD patients about their diagnosis, prognosis, and all treatment options.

Recommendation No. 3: Give all patients with AKI, stage 5 CKD, or ESRD an estimate of prognosis specific to their overall condition.

Recommendation No. 4: Institute advance care planning.

Recommendation No. 5: If appropriate, forgo (withhold initiating or withdraw ongoing) dialysis for patients with AKI, CKD, or ESRD in certain, well-defined situations.

Recommendation No. 6: Consider forgoing dialysis for AKI, CKD, or ESRD patients who have a very poor prognosis or for whom dialysis cannot be provided safely.

Recommendation No. 7: Consider a time-limited trial of dialysis for patients requiring dialysis, but who have an uncertain prognosis, or for whom a consensus cannot be reached about providing dialysis.

Recommendation No. 8: Establish a systematic due process approach for conflict resolution if there is disagreement about what decision should be made with regard to dialysis.

Recommendation No. 9: To improve patient-centered outcomes, offer palliative care services and interventions to all AKI, CKD, and ESRD patients who suffer from burdens of their disease.

Recommendation No. 10: Use a systematic approach to communicate about diagnosis, prognosis, treatment options, and goals of care.

The ICU team speaks with the patient and family, and subsequently agrees that transition to comfort care is consistent with the patient's wishes. He is prescribed medicine to be given as needed for any pain, anxiety, or shortness of breath. CRRT is discontinued, pressors are slowly weaned, and he dies 48 hours later in his ICU room with his siblings at his bedside.

Take-Away Points
1. Patients with ESRD have high mortality, higher even than many cancers, especially with advanced age and comorbidities. It is important to be able to formulate prognosis.
2. Hope and worry statements can simultaneously align yourself with patients/families while pivoting to consideration of less favorable clinical outcomes.
3. The PERSON mnemonic is a useful framework for guiding a person-informed goals-of-care discussion.
4. Acknowledging and supporting colleague distress with difficult care decisions is integral to the practice of medicine.

References

1. Davison SN. End-of-life care preferences and needs: perceptions of patients with chronic kidney disease. Clin J Am Soc Nephrol. 2010;5:195–204.
2. Davison SN, et al. Nephrologists' reported preparedness for end-of-life decision-making. Clin J Am Soc Nephrol. 2006;1:1256–62.

3. Schell JO, et al. Communication skills training for dialysis decision-making and end-of-life care in nephrology. Clin J Am Soc Nephrol. 2013;8:675–80.
4. United States Renal Data System. Annual Data Report: Epidemiology of Kidney Disease in the United States. Bethesda, MD: National Institutes of Health, National Institute of Diabetes and Digestive and Kidney Diseases; 2018, 2018
5. O'Hare AM. Palliative and end-of-life care in patients with kidney disease. USRDS special study on palliative and end-of-life care. https://www.usrds.org/2014/pres/ASN_usrds_OHare_Presented.pdf.
6. Edmonds KP, Toluwalase AA, Cain J, Yeung HN, Thornberry K. Establishing goals of care at any stage of illness: The PERSON mnemonic. J Palliat Med. 2014 Oct;17(10):1087.
7. Moss AH. Revised Dialysis clinical practice guideline promotes more informed decision-making. CJASN. 2010;5(12):2380–3.

Chapter 17
Teaching Learners How to Approach Family Decisions as a Process

Alan Garber

Case Introduction

Mrs. B is an 89-year-old widow with advanced Parkinson's disease, dementia, and heart failure and is admitted to the ICU for septic shock secondary to a UTI. She is intubated, on several vasopressors, with worsening oliguria, and is sedated to RASS-4 for agitation and ventilator dyssynchrony. She is full code, without prior advance directive. Multiple family members have been at bedside daily. Per the charge nurse, the family "just doesn't get it." Multiple nursing, respiratory therapist, and resident notes indicate a strong suggestion for comfort care.

Usual Approach

Mrs. B is continued on antibiotics, ventilator, and pressor support. Over the next week, she continues to deteriorate. The resident provides thorough daily updates to her family; however, he is bewildered why they never get closer to making a decision. Her family identifies a handful of clinical staff whom they trust as their advocates. Eventually, the patient's profound lactic acidosis leads to arrhythmia, cardiac arrest, and an unsuccessful prolonged resuscitation.

A. Garber (✉)
Department of Medicine, Mary Imogene Bassett Hospital, Cooperstown, NY, USA

© Springer Nature Switzerland AG 2020

K. Aberger, D. Wang (eds.), *Palliative Skills for Frontline Clinicians*,
https://doi.org/10.1007/978-3-030-44414-3_17

Palliative Approach

During your morning rounds, you invite Mrs. B's family to join your team. As the attending, you set expectations for both the family and your team: "At various times we will ask for your input and we will also explain our thoughts and plans in plain language. If at the end of rounds there needs to be further discussion, we will find dedicated time for a longer family meeting in our conference room." Your resident reviews her evolving clinical picture. Her family listens intently and asks a handful of questions.

Your resident then thoughtfully asks the family what name to best address the patient. "Dora," they say. Your resident then asks, "When Dora was healthier in the past, did she ever talk about what she would want her care to be like if she ever became this ill?" Abruptly, her youngest daughter angrily accuses your team, "You're trying to get us to pull the plug on her, aren't you?" Your resident appears uncomfortable. Sensing tension, you reassure them: "We are here with only one job: to give your mom the best care possible. We just want to learn more about her to provide a human side to our practice of medicine. May I suggest we meet again later this afternoon to continue our conversation?" They agree to meet at 2 pm.

Afterwards, you notice your resident looks fine but ask him anyway how he felt during that interaction. He admits, "I get frustrated when patients and families direct anger at me." He did not always feel this way, but as he has increased his knowledge and personal sacrifice in his training, he feels insulted when his commitment isn't valued. You create a teaching moment to share your own experience in managing anger.

Box 17.1 Responding to Anger

For many clinicians, anger is one of the most, if not the absolute most, difficult emotion to receive. Responses can include reciprocated anger, defensiveness, anxiety, fear, hurt, or any combination of these. Our response tends reflect our personalities and personal experiences receiving anger in the past. For families, it is important to remember that anger is often a displaced secondary emotion. There is a greater underlying driver: fear of losing their loved one, powerlessness from a loss of sense of control, guilt, or regret from unfinished business with their loved one, etc.

Effective response to anger includes:

- Silence
- Gentle exploration: "I sense you're really angry about how the you feel your mother's care has been handled."
- Admission and redirection: "You're right. I don't think there's anything I could say to justify how long you have waited. You have my full attention and care now. How can I best help?"

Prior to the afternoon family meeting, you notice that the bedside nurse has built great rapport with the family. You ask her for her assessment of the situation. She shares "They're just really struggling. But I told them the blood pressure is a little better today and I backed off the levophed a bit, and that cheered them up." You recognize how information can be both delivered and received with varying positivity. You also worry that Dora's family may be receiving mixed messages given how they've seemed hot and cold to various staff. As always, you invite the bedside nurse to the meeting today to ensure consistency in messaging.

Prior to the family meeting, you premeet with your resident and team. You ask the resident his approach to leading this meeting. He states, "I don't think they're ready to talk about code status, but I think I can at least get a DNR today." You remind him that while code status is a critical element for ICU teams, it is more effectively addressed when couched at the end of a broader goals-of-care conversation as a recommendation than an open-ended floating question. Your resident responds, "But nobody wants to code this woman." You agree, and additionally say that it is may be more traumatizing for Dora's family to weigh this question de novo than to be gradually moved through the acceptance of this being the end of Dora's life. Moreover, she is already on several forms of life support, and a few rounds of CPR and medications would not make a significant difference. An ICU priority is not necessarily a family priority.

You propose instead a different approach to the family meeting, and lay out some ground rules (Table 17.1):

Your resident gathers the case manager, social worker, bedside nurse, charge nurse, and cardiology and nephrology consultants. He will lead the meeting, with you jumping in as necessary, and may ask several of them for their perspectives at different points. He reviews the medical assessment and asks for any additional input. After reviewing the staff's recent interactions with family, everybody agrees that the best care possible for the patient necessitates supporting her family by establishing trust and consistency. There will be no discussions regarding code status or comfort care. The primary objective is to align ourselves with them. Lastly, he thanks them in advance for what he anticipates will be an hour of their time.

Table 17.1 Preplanning the ICU family meeting

Who will lead	Leader can be ICU team, specialty team, or nonclinical person with strong rapport (e.g., chaplain). Often the intensivist will start the meeting and then delegate specific roles/content to other parties.
Who needs to attend from clinical teams	Ensure agreement of clinical opinions especially when intermediary surgical interventions are available. Can be frustrating for families to hear different assessments from different teams (e.g., "her [organ] is getting stronger").
Who needs to attend from family	Do not assume that the people at the bedside are the people that need, or even should, be present. If possible, have the patient designate.
Meeting expectations/ agenda	Establish agreement of the objectives which may include breaking bad news, understanding quality of life goals, limit setting on escalation of care, and/or clarifying code status. A successful meeting, especially with a defensive family, can involve nothing more than rapport building and exploration.
Meeting duration	Prepare all parties with an internal timeline which allows them to rearrange their speaking order should they have to exit early.

Your resident asks other meeting members to help bring extra chairs to the conference room. Your resident begins the meeting with introductions. He lays out what he hopes to discuss, and then asks them if there are priorities on their minds as well. The same daughter from before says, "I want to know why some people are telling us she's getting better, and others make it sounds like we need to make funeral arrangements. Are you all talking to each other? What's really going on?" Your resident is more prepared this time: "I hear your concern, and it's a fair one. Thanks for being open with us. I can't imagine how frustrating that is. Dora's care is complex, and we have complex clinical perspectives ourselves. My hope for today's meeting is by gathering her experts here all together so we can all be on the same page and you can hear it from the source." She appreciates this, uncrossing her arms, nodding, and now leaning into his direction.

Your resident then says something that changes the entire atmosphere of the room: "We are not asking for any decisions today." It feels like a great weight has been lifted in the room, and everybody sits up straighter. One nephew says, "Thank you for saying that, we feel like we've been backed into a corner these last few days." Several clinical team members offer empathetic responses and reassurance. This creates an opening for more dialogue. He asks more about Dora: "In the ICU we only see your loved one in a limited way. Tell us about her."

They begin to tell her story. How she met her husband. How she was a beloved English teacher. How she and their father before he died would visit England (she loved modern British fiction). They get quite emotional and state that it is so hard to see her in this state in the ICU. She and her husband were schoolteachers and had three daughters (all in the area) and eight grandchildren. He died a few years ago.

Several times your resident indicates he wants to move forward in the conversation, but you give him subtle cutes to wait. You allow family ample space to tell her story, recognizing this is part of the grieving process. Then you nod to the resident, who asks, "And now, looking back at just the last year, how have things been Dora?"

There is a collective sigh from family. They share that she is now fully care dependent at the nursing facility and bedbound. She soils the bed daily, and they feel she has lost the tremendous dignity with which she lived life and raised them. Over the past 3 months, it seems that she no longer even recognizes her daughters. One son says, "We know she is nearing the end of her life; we're doing our best to keep her comfortable." Family members take turns hand-feeding her meals. They play music for her that she and her husband loved. And mostly they sit quietly with her.

Your social worker chimes in and says, "What has been your source of strength through all of these changes?" The family shares about how the patient raised all of them and has been a matriarch. "She gave up so much to take care of us, so now we need to do right by her."

Your resident continues on, "I agree with you that Dora is likely nearing the end of her life, despite our best efforts. She could not have made it to this day without the love and care you have been providing her. Please trust that every person here from our teams will be doing our best to care for Dora." Dora's family appreciate that he acknowledges their commitment. Recognizing the rapport your team has now built, you conclude this meeting with: "I will make a commitment to you all that we will partner with you every step forward on this journey, wherever it leads." Dora's family hugs you and your resident as the meeting concludes.

Afterwards, you debrief the meeting with all parties involved, and ask everyone to provide feedback to your resident.

Box 17.2 Teaching Communication by Giving Feedback

Learners improve communication skills as much by receiving feedback as they do by directly leading family meetings. Although everybody is eager to disperse after a long meeting, do not forego this important last step, which can be abbreviated if needed.

Giving feedback must be both intentional and focused. Intentionality primes the learner to pay attention and reflect: "Let's take a few minutes. I'd like for us all to give you feedback on how that went." Helpful feedback must be focused. Instead, have all parties share one observation of what the learner executed well. And then ask the learner what is one thing they would like to do differently next time. If they are unable to identify a goal, provide them one and one only. It is not helpful to identify several learning goals, which are too overwhelming to implement all at once. Some learners are hypercritical of themselves and will gravitate toward this habit; streamline their attention for step-wise growth.

Over the next 2 days, your team continues to round together with the family in the morning. The family learns that Dora unfortunately has progressed into multiorgan failure. She is becoming edematous, has developed shock liver, has a rising lactate, and now has ARDS. With sedation turned off, she remains RASS-5. The family has been keeping vigil. They see and understand these ominous changes.

The next day, the family requests another family meeting and asks for your resident by name to be there. During your premeeting, your resident reviews that he has spoken with several family members individually over the last 2 days and they appreciate that the ICU has "done everything they can for Dora." The tension and sense of mistrust has melted away. You remind your resident to focus on big picture goals first, and now get mired down with small decisions like code status at the beginning.

The family meeting begins. After your resident provides a brief medical update, then asks an open-ended question, "How are you all feeling about Dora?" There is a long pause. Her youngest daughter begins to cry. Your team remains silent and waits. She gathers herself and states how hard that this has been but that she has been so grateful for your team's openness. She says, "We've fulfilled our responsibility to her. We can't keep her here, that's only for us and not for her. It's time for us to let her go. She's going to be with her husband. We will see her again." Other family members echo in agreement. Your resident makes a recommendation for comfort care and compassionate extubation to which they readily agree. He follows this up with a brief recommendation for code status change: "And when the time comes and she has died a natural death, we will let her body be." All are in agreement.

Your resident is amazed at how this structured approach over the last few days actually made these conversations easier, and likely less drawn out, than they might have been. You further add that while it is great for our jobs to be easier, the most important thing is the family's memory of these days, and the legacy they will carry with them forever.

Later that day, Dora is extubated and dies peacefully with her family by her side. Following Dora's death, her daughter pulls you aside and says, "I'm going to share with your resident too but I wanted you to hear this from me: He is going to be a wonderfully kind doctor. He should know this meant the world to us."

Take-Away Points
1. Equally important to family meetings are the family interactions occurring during regular care and team rounds. These are opportunities to learn background information, explore family dynamics, build rapport, and augment topics discussed during larger meetings.
2. Responding to anger is challenging for many clinicians. It helps to remember that anger is often a displaced secondary emotion which may overlay fear, helplessness, guilt, or regret.
3. A structured approach to effective family meetings is built upon systematic preplanning.
4. Feedback to learners augments their experiential learning from leading meetings. Feedback should be intentional and focused.
5. Silence can often be more powerful than words. Allow families space to process their feelings, express uncertainties, and grieve, before asking for decisions.

Part III
Surgery

Chapter 18
Trach/PEG Consult in the ICU

Christine Toevs

Case Introduction

Mrs. V is a 74-year-old woman admitted from home with respiratory failure secondary to a COPD exacerbation. She has been intubated for longer than 2 weeks. She also has stable coronary disease and insulin-dependent diabetes. You are consulted to place a tracheostomy and a gastrostomy tube (trach/PEG), so she can be transferred to a long-term acute care hospital (LTACH) for long-term care and continued attempts to wean off the ventilator. She has mild delirium and cannot participate in her own decision-making at this time.

Usual Approach

A trach/PEG allows for transfer and placement in an LTACH for continued weaning attempts. The procedures are not technically difficult, both can be done at beside in the ICU or in the operating room, and take about an hour. You speak with family, explain the procedures, and have them sign a consent form. The procedures are successful, and the patient is transferred to an LTACH several days later. She is readmitted several times over the next few months for further COPD exacerbations, ventilator-associated pneumonia, and decubitus ulcers, and she ultimately dies 8 months later. She never is weaned off of the ventilator.

C. Toevs (✉)
Terre Haute Regional Hospital, Terre Haute, IN, USA
e-mail: ctoevs@pghphysician.com

© Springer Nature Switzerland AG 2020
K. Aberger, D. Wang (eds.), *Palliative Skills for Frontline Clinicians*,
https://doi.org/10.1007/978-3-030-44414-3_18

Palliative Approach

You delve deeper into her history. She has a history of COPD and has required three admissions for noninvasive ventilation in the past several months. She is on home oxygen.

Although the surgeon is often consulted as a technician in these clinical scenarios, there is still an obligation to explain the procedure and the outcomes to the patient. Although the procedure is technically feasible with minimal risk, there are long-term consequences of which they should be informed. The family often expects the patient to "get better" after the procedure. However, trach/PEG does not "treat" the patient's disease or change outcome. The trach/PEG will allow for the patient to be placed in a long-term ventilator weaning hospital (LTACH). For patients with chronic critical illness, and prolonged mechanical ventilation (a form of chronic critical illness), the odds of independent living at 1 year is 11%. Over half die within a year, and of those who survive, most require long-term nursing home placement. Very few patients wean from the ventilator or recover enough for rehab treatment [1-5].

Box 18.1 Paint a Realistic Picture Using Language of Functional Outcomes

Managing expectations in this case are important. Telling the family that surgery does not change outcome, and only allows for placement options, is critical to the informed consent process. Discussion of long-term functional recovery is very important to the families and, if able, the patient. Elaborate on what functional baseline would merit a meaningful quality of life to help you phrase your recommendations on whether these interventions will meet those goals of care.

Your first step is to meet with the consulting physician to ask what their expectations are regarding this patient's long-term outcome. "Do you expect her to wean from the ventilator? How significant is her COPD? How have your conversations been with the family? Have you addressed code status and long-term outcomes? May I do so in the context of a trach/PEG? Would you be okay if the family decides on comfort measures and end-of-life care? Do you want to be there when I speak with the family and address goals of care?"

Box 18.2 Optimism Bias in Prognosis Affects Physicians and Surrogates

Doctors significantly overestimate survival. Studies have shown that the expected prognosis did not match the observed outcome in at least 36% of patients, and 99% of the time that was due to over-optimism on the part of the physician [6]. Surrogates also have inaccurate expectations about prognosis, and two-thirds triangulate physician communication with their own values, beliefs, and experiences.

The physician tells you that her COPD is end stage, and she has been on home oxygen for a year. She has had multiple admissions for COPD exacerbations in the past several years, with several in the last few months. The intensivist tells you that he doesn't expect her to wean from the vent, but the family "isn't ready to pull the plug."

You make time to meet with the family in order to provide an explanation of the long-term consequences of a trach/PEG. You meet with the children and the spouse, who is in poor health himself, and defers decisions to the adult children. You ask the bedside nurse and the ICU social worker to be present. This conversation takes about 30 minutes.

Box 18.3 Don't Rush It
Plan on these conversations taking 30–45 minutes. Sit in the ICU conference room with the family and staff and give them your full attention, since they often perceive doctors as too busy to talk with them.

The conversation proceeds:

You   "Your wife/mother seems very weak to me. What do you know about her current medical problems and time in the hospital and ICU?"

Family "Yes, she is sick, but we think she will get better and go home and a trach/PEG is going to help her get there. She is a fighter."

You   "It seems she has had a really tough time of it the past few years. Tell me how she has been doing."

Family "Yes, it has been very hard. She has been in the hospital many times and each time we take her home, she seems weaker and weaker. This last time a few months ago, she never really bounced back."

You   "Has she been losing weight? Does she get out of the house much? How is her memory? What does she like to do? Is she able to do those things? How much do you have to help her with dressing, bathing, cooking, getting around? What makes her happy?"

Talking about her life the past few years appears to help the family, as it allows them to express what they have seen, what she is been going through, and the difficulties on them. They talk about her life, her independence, her stubbornness, her appetite for life, and her love of her home and her family. They also talk about the impact of her illness on her the last few years, especially recently. They describe her decline, limitations, and functional changes. You give the family time to talk over this information and process their experiences.

You then lay out the best case/worst case scenario [7].

You   "Wow, she sounds like a really cool lady. It seems like it has been a rough time recently. I have been asked to place a trach/PEG in your mother and I want to talk about what that will look like. Seeing your mother for the first time, it looks like she is really doing poorly and is slowly dying. Let's talk best case, worst case.

Best case, of course, is that she completely recovers and goes home and does great, but that isn't going to happen. Your mother is on full-life support. The ventilator and tube feeds are life-support and machines are keeping her alive. Families tend to think that doing these procedures will help their loved ones get better. They don't. This surgery won't help her come off the ventilator, but rather allow us to place her in a long-term ventilator weaning hospital. The goal will be to get your mom off the ventilator, but given her decline in the past several years, and especially in the past few months, it is not likely. That means she will live in a nursing home for the rest of her life.

Worst case is that she dies, but in some cases, there are things that can be worse than death for the patient and family. The trach/PEG is going to be permanent. With a trach and on the ventilator, she cannot talk. As her body continues to decline, she will have a variety of complications. I'm not sure which ones, but the common ones are pneumonia, frequent readmissions to the hospital, stroke, heart attack, GI bleed, bedsores, and ultimately death. I know you want her to go home and get well, but that really isn't going to happen here, even with surgery. You said being with her grandchildren was very important to her. They can come visit her, but she won't be able to pick them up or talk with them. Even if she comes off the ventilator, she will need a nursing home for the remainder of her life. She will need help dressing, bathing, brushing her teeth, and feeding herself."

Box 18.4 Be Precise with Language

Families tend to understand the significance of the decisions to be made when defined in the context of what is important to their loved one. Using the term "life support" is critical. Some families may not realize that the ventilator is a form of life-support. Even fewer recognize the same for pressors and artificial nutrition, which are less visible and palpable. Always include "she is on life-support" and "the machines are keeping her alive." Avoid gentler euphemisms such as "the machine is helping her to breathe" or "the nutrition will help her body get stronger."

You continue on, "Given what you have told me about her, how would she feel about living like this?" One of her daughters says bluntly, "mom would never want to live like this." A son cuts her off and says, "she wouldn't want to give up! She will come off the machine! You will see!" and then he starts crying and abruptly leaves the meeting. The remaining siblings talk about how close they are, he lives with her and is having the hardest time watching her decline and suffer. They believe he doesn't want to see her suffer any more either, and they plan to have a family meeting among themselves that night to discuss their mother's care. They are grateful to you for being direct and admit that they "knew this was coming, but didn't want to admit it [8, 9]."

Box 18.5 Emotions Are Necessary
Families tend to understand the significance of the decisions to be made, but when they are defined in the context of families there may be complicated dynamics. It takes skill to manage a family meeting and to allow everyone to be heard. Learning how to recognize and respond to emotion is critical. Emotional processing is crucial to making these decisions, and the showing of emotion is almost always a good sign.

Case Conclusion

When you regroup with the family the next day, the discussion starts much the same way. "How can I help you? What questions can I answer for you?" They ask their options are if they do not choose the trach/PEG. "We will stop the machines and allow a natural death. We will focus entirely on her comfort and make sure she isn't suffering, but we won't do anything to hasten her death. I don't know exactly when she will die, but it may be a few hours to a few days. In any case, we will keep her comfortable and you can be with her."

The family reports that they spoke all together the night before and decided on comfort care. They say that she would never want this and would want to die with dignity. The son is still tearful, but appears at peace. You reassure them that based on what they told you the day before about their mother, and what you know about her medical condition, that they are doing the right thing.

Box 18.6 Putting the Patient First
Many families have fear or guilt over making this decision, and struggle when there are no explicit advanced directives or prior conversations. Helping the family anchor the medical information in the context of who the patient is as a person and how they would feel in this situation helps them navigate these complex decisions and step outside of themselves to put the patient first.

Take-Away Points
1. Use the terms "life-support" and "being kept alive on machines."
2. Emphasize that trach/PEG do not change outcome or recovery, but instead only allow for placement outside of the hospital, first in a ventilatory weaning hospital, then in a nursing home.
3. Have family tell their story sharing their perception of her functional decline before she went into the hospital and her subsequent time there Recognize and acknowledge emotion.
4. Encourage them to speak for her, what is important in her life, and what she would say – try and separate that from their own emotions.

References

1. Bice T, Nelson JE, Carson SS. To trach or not to trach: uncertainty in the care of the chronically critically ill. Semin Respir Crit Care Med. 2015;36:851–8.
2. Carson SS, Bach PB, Brzozowski L, Leff A. Outcomes after long-term acute care: an analysis of 133 mechanically ventilated patients. Am J Respir Crit Care Med. 1999;159:1568–73.
3. Chiarchiaro J, Buddadhumaruk P, Arnold RM, et al. Quality of communication in the ICU and surrogate's understanding of prognosis. Crit Care Med. 2015;43:542–8.
4. Damuth E, Mitchell JA, Bartock JL, et al. Long-term survival of critically ill patients treated with prolonged mechanical ventilation: a systematic review and meta-analysis. Lancet Respir Med. 2015;3:544–53.
5. Kruser JM, Taylor LJ, Campbell TC, et al. "Best care/worst case": training surgeon to use a novel communication tool for high-risk acute surgical problems. J Pain Symptom Manag. 2017;53:711–9.
6. Raiten JM, Meuman MD. "If I had only known" – on choice and uncertainty in the ICU. NEJM. 2012;367:1779–81.
7. Ruggiero RM. Chronic critical illness: the limbo between life and death. Am J Med Sci. 2018;355:286–92.
8. Soliman IW, Cremer OL, deLange DW, et al. The ability of intensive care physicians to estimate long-term prognosis in survivors of critical illness. J Crit Care. 2018;43:148–55.
9. Unroe M, Kahn JM, Carson SS, et al. One-year trajectories of care and resource utilization for recipients of prolonged mechanical ventilation. Ann Intern Med. 2010;153:167–75.

Chapter 19
Rescinding DNR Orders in the Operating Room

Melissa Red Hoffman

Case Introduction

Mrs. Brown, an 82-year-old female, presents with a large bowel obstruction secondary to cecal volvulus. She has a medical history of COPD (on 2 L of home oxygen) and atrial fibrillation (rate controlled with metoprolol, anticoagulated with coumadin) as well as a remote history of a stroke with minimal right-sided deficits. She has a surgical history of a hysterectomy. She currently lives alone and remains active in her community. She arrives at the hospital without any advance directives.

You meet with Mrs. Brown and her daughter Jane in the emergency department. Based on your physical exam as well as the labs and imaging obtained by the ED physician, you explain to her and her daughter that you recommend an operation.

Usual Approach

You obtain consent, but do not address advance directives, as no one took the time to locate them in the electronic medical record (EMR). You proceed immediately to the operating room, as this is an emergent situation. (If you do find evidence of DNR, it would be automatically rescinded during surgery and likely not addressed afterwards.) She develops complications and is taken back to the OR. She is not able to be extubated after the second operation, and the family grapples with the decision to remove life support. You are frustrated with the family's inability to let go and offer a trach/PEG for long-term nursing home placement. After days of family indecision, you finally consult palliative care.

M. R. Hoffman (✉)
Department of Surgery, Mission Hospital, Asheville, NC, USA

© Springer Nature Switzerland AG 2020
K. Aberger, D. Wang (eds.), *Palliative Skills for Frontline Clinicians*,
https://doi.org/10.1007/978-3-030-44414-3_19

Palliative Approach

You delve deeper into the patient's history and comb through the EMR. Mrs. Brown was last hospitalized approximately 6 months ago following a ground level fall that resulted in a small subdural hematoma. During that admission, she was seen by palliative care to discuss the risks and benefits of continuing coumadin. At that time, the palliative care team reviewed her advance care planning documents and confirmed that her daughter Jane was her healthcare power of attorney (HCPOA). The palliative care team also filled out a POLST (Physician Orders for Life-Sustaining Treatment) form with the patient and scanned it into the electronic medical record (EMR).

You review her current workup as well as notes from her last hospitalization. You review her advance directives including her POLST form. On the POLST form, Mrs. Brown indicated that she is a Do-Not-Resuscitate (DNR) and that she would prefer only Limited Additional Interventions.

You print out a copy of the POLST and review it with Mrs. Brown and Jane. In this instance, Mrs. Brown, despite filling out the form just 6 months ago, is now uncertain about what she wants to do. She is now considering surgery. Given this, you utilize the Best Case/Worst Case (BC/WC) framework to guide Mrs. Brown and Jane in their decision-making process [1].

Box 19.1 Best Case/Worst Case
Rather than present risk and benefits of surgery using statistical statements, or focusing exclusively on simplified clinical outcomes (e.g., full recovery, death), paint the functional outcomes and medical experiences that could arise with or without surgery.

You present Mrs. Brown with two options – surgery or supportive care – and then go on to describe the best case, the worst case, and the most likely outcome for each choice. In the first option, surgery, the best case is a short surgery after which Mrs. Brown is extubated, has a relatively quick return of bowel function with a 4- to 5-day hospital stay and a discharge back to home. The worst case is a longer surgery secondary to scar tissue; an inability to be extubated with a prolonged ICU stay; complications including pneumonia, anastomotic leak, or DVT formation; and eventual death in the ICU. Lastly, the most likely outcome is a short surgery with an admission to the ICU secondary to underlying pulmonary disease, possible pneumonia, and discharge to a skilled nursing facility.

You continue the BC/WC framework by then presenting the second option, supportive care. The best case is that Mrs. Brown will be discharged to home with hospice, remain conscious for several days so that she can spend time with her family, have good pain control, and die in her own bed. The worst case is that she will die in the hospital before her family has a chance to arrive. Finally, the most likely outcome is that she will quickly become septic and have altered mental status, be unable to speak with her family, and die either in the hospital or in an inpatient hospice facility.

Mrs. Brown decides to pursue surgery. You feel another conversation to explore code status is necessary to clarify status during the perioperative period. You explain to Mrs. Brown that she can choose whether to uphold or suspend her DNR order during the perioperative period.

> **Box 19.2 Do Not Resuscitate Orders in the Operating Room**
> The American College of Surgeons, the American Society of Anesthesiologists, and the Association of Operating Room Nurses have all published statements regarding DNR orders in the operating room [2–4]. The American College of Surgeons recommends a policy of "required reconsideration" of the DNR order. During "required reconsideration," the surgeon, the anesthesiologist, the patient, and their surrogate decision makers engage in a discussion of the risks and benefits of surgery, the patient's goals of care, and the various options for treatment of life-threatening problems which can occur during surgery [2].

Case Continued

Mrs. Brown chooses to rescind her DNR during the perioperative period. Her daughter Jane is visibly upset that her mother keeps "changing her mind." You know there is no formal definition of the "perioperative period." Therefore, you along with Mrs. Brown, Jane, and the anesthesiologist have a discussion to define when the DNR order will once again be valid and document this decision in the EMR.

Furthermore, because you know Mrs. Brown is at high risk for decompensation after surgery, you also take the time to discuss potential complications and to explore some decisions that Jane, as her HCPOA may be asked to make in the future. For example, you discuss the possible need for prolonged ventilatory support given the history of COPD and clarify that Mrs. Brown would not want a tracheostomy placed if she were unable to be weaned from the ventilator after 2 weeks.

Lastly, you note that Jane is visibly distressed that her mother has "changed her mind." While Mrs. Brown currently retains the capacity to make complex medical and Jane's opinion is of no legal consequence, palliative medicine is dedicated to the care of both the patient and the family. Therefore, you acknowledge Jane's distress and take the time to explain to her that studies have shown that older patients with advanced illness tend to change their preferences regarding life-sustaining treatment, often in unpredictable ways [5]. You involve the palliative care team early to help the family through this decision-making process.

You take Mrs. Brown to surgery and perform a right hemicolectomy with a primary ileocolic anastomosis. She does well throughout the surgery and is extubated postoperatively. On postoperative day 4, she develops a hospital-acquired pneumonia. She requires high-flow nasal cannula (HFNC) for 48 hours and remarks, "I hate that thing in my nose." On postoperative day 8, during an extended coughing episode during the night, she feels a sudden "pop." On rounds the next morning, you confirm that she has experienced a fascial dehiscence.

Before discussing your findings and your proposed plan, you ask Mrs. Brown if she would like her family present. Mrs. Brown requests that you call her daughter Jane and place her on speaker phone so that she can hear your findings and proposed plan.

You start by reviewing the events that have occurred during the past week. You acknowledge that "this Mrs. Brown" is not the same patient whom you operated on a week ago. Mrs. Brown now has already had one operation and is currently being treated for pneumonia. She has also experienced a functional decline associated with being hospitalized. You explain that you will not know exactly what procedure needs to be performed until you are in the operating room. In order to further assist Mrs. Brown and Jane with their decision-making, as well as to set reasonable expectations, you have used the American College of Surgeons National Surgical Quality Improvement Program (ACS NSQIP) Surgical Risk Calculator to estimate the chance of multiple postoperative complications including the risks of cardiac complication; renal failure; need to return to OR; discharge to a nursing facility; and death [6, 7]. You subsequently share these with Mrs. Brown (Table 19.1).

Table 19.1 American College of Surgeons Surgical Risk Calculator Example

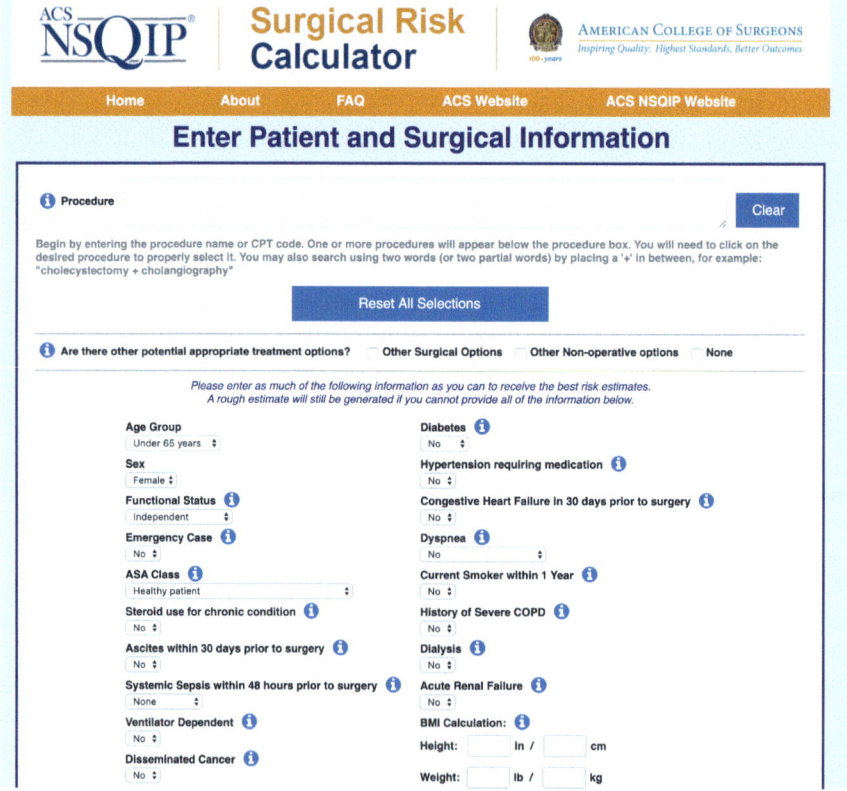

Copyright American College of Surgeons National Quality Improvement Program. Please note that this data collection page is preceded by an introductory page, including permitted use and disclaimer, and followed by pages which provide results and options for reporting them

Mrs. Brown decides she wants to proceed with surgery. Before obtaining consent, you once again discuss Mrs. Brown's advance directives and ask whether she wants to uphold or rescind her DNR order during the perioperative period. Based on her previous POLST form, you also clarify whether she would be willing to remain intubated after the procedure (given her already tenuous respiratory status).

In this instance, based on her experiences in the past week, Mrs. Brown chooses to keep her DNR order in place during surgery. After further discussion, Mrs. Brown also clarifies that she wants to be extubated after the case and that she does not want to be intubated in the case of further respiratory decline. She is not willing to live or suffer with further incapacitation. Per hospital policy, she is asked to sign a separate consent indicating these choices. Both you and the anesthesiologist document this conversation in the EMR as well.

You take Mrs. Brown back to the operating room. During induction, she vomits and has a likely aspiration event. You explore the abdomen and confirm that there is no evidence of infection and that the anastomosis is intact. You repair the fascial dehiscence and anesthesia is able to extubate Mrs. Brown at the end of the case. However, she requires HFNC overnight, and the next day her respiratory status continues to decline, leading to increasing oxygen requirements.

Throughout the day, the nurse pages you several times to discuss the plan for the patient. When you round again in the afternoon, Mrs. Brown is minimally responsive and tachypneic with an oxygen saturation of 86% on 100% HFNC. You find both the bedside nurse and the charge nurse discussing the patient; the bedside nurse is visibly upset.

Because one of the central tenets of palliative care is caring for the patient, the family, and the entire care team, you approach the charge nurse and the bedside nurse and engage in discussion. You acknowledge that the nurse appears distressed and you ask her if she would like to discuss this further. She says that it appears that Mrs. Brown likely has a reversible condition that may respond to several days of antibiotics and mechanical ventilation. You confirm that this may be true but also review that Mrs. Brown specifically told both you and the anesthesiologist that she is not willing to live with the further incapacitation that is inevitable with further aggressive measures such as intubation. You also acknowledge that it must be very difficult for her to watch Mrs. Brown rapidly declining and to feel like there is nothing she can do to improve the situation.

You call Jane and let her know that her mother has continued to decline throughout the day, despite maximum oxygen therapy. You explain that given her mother's expressed wishes, you are not planning to intubate her and that you think she will likely only worsen in the next few hours. Jane asks if there is anything else to do.

You continue to use your primary palliative care skills and explain to Jane that because Mrs. Brown was clear about her goals, the best course of action at this point is to transition to comfort care. You explain that this would entail starting an opioid to relieve dyspnea and then stopping the HFNC. Jane expresses concern that without oxygen, her mother will suffocate as she has been on home oxygen for years. You take the time to explain that continuing HFNC may actually prolong the dying process [8]. When Jane asks you how long her mother will survive, you respond that it is difficult to know for certain, but that she probably has hours to days left to live.

You initiate the comfort care order set for Mrs. Brown. Once she appears comfortable, you remove the HFNC. Ten hours later, she dies with Jane at the bedside.

Take-Away Points
1. Regardless of their prior advance directives, patients may – and have the right to – change their preferences as they experience changes in their health. Therefore, it is recommended that physicians take the time to review a patient's advance directives (including living will, code status, and POLST form) when the patient transfers from one care setting to another and when there is a substantial change in the patient's medical condition [9].
2. Multiple societies, including the American College of Surgeons, the American Society of Anesthesiologists, and the Association of Operating Room Nurses have all published statements regarding the continuation of DNR orders in the operating room. The American College of Surgeons Statement on Advance Directives by Patients specifically states, "policies that lead to either automatic enforcement of all DNR orders or to disregarding or automatically cancelling such orders do not sufficiently support a patient's right to self-determination" [2].
3. The Best Case/Worst Case framework is a crucial discussion tool meant to support shared decision-making when speaking with families about difficult choices. Use the ACS NSQIP Surgical Risk Calculator to aid in prognostication. Prognostication is often the key to managing expectations and making decisions.
4. Our colleagues – nurses, residents, any other members of the healthcare team – may need extra support and education when dealing with cases like this. They often cause distress in colleagues that may inadvertently negatively impact the patient and family.
5. High-flow nasal cannula may prolong the dying process. Because it is another form of noninvasive positive pressure ventilation (albeit more comfortable than BiPAP), physicians should be thoughtful about whether or not to offer it to patients who may already be in the dying process, and should also be thoughtful about when to discontinue it [8].

References

1. Taylor LJ, Nabozny MJ, Steffens NM, Tucholka JL, Brasel KJ, Johnson SK, et al. A framework to improve surgeon communication in high-stakes surgical decisions. JAMA Surg. 2017;152(6):531–41.
2. American College of Surgeons. Statement on advance directives by patients: do not resuscitate in the operating room. 2014. https://www.facs.org/about-acs/statements/19-advance-directives. Accessed on 15 Jan 2019.
3. American Society of Anesthesiologists. Ethical guidelines for the anesthesia care of patients with do-not-resuscitate orders or other directives that limit treatment. 2018. https://www.asahq.

org/~/media/sites/asahq/files/public/resources/standards-guidelines/ethical-guidelines-for-the-anesthesia-care-of-patients.pdf. Accessed on 15 Jan 2019.
4. Association of Perioperative Registered Nurses. AORN position statement on perioperative care of Patients with do-not-resuscitate or allow natural death orders. 2014. https://www.aorn. org/-/media/aorn/guidelines/position-statements/posstat-dnr-w.pdf. Accessed on 15 Jan 2019.
5. Fried TR, O'Leary J, Van Ness P, Fraenkel L. Inconsistency over time in the preferences of older persons with advanced illness for life-sustaining treatment. J Am Geriatr Soc. 2007;55:1007–14. Accessed on 15 Jan 2019.
6. ACS Risk Calculator – Home Page. https://riskcalculator.facs.org/RiskCalculator/index.jsp. Accessed on 15 Jan 2019.
7. Bilimoria KY, Liu Y, Paruch JL, Zhou L, Kmiecik TE, Ko CY, et al. Development and evaluation of the universal ACS NSQIP surgical risk calculator: a decision aid and informed consent tool for patients and surgeons. J Am Coll Surg. 2013;217:833–42.
8. Shah N, Mehta Z, Mehta Y. Fast facts and concepts #330: high-flow nasal cannula oxygen therapy in palliative care. 2018. https://www.mypcnow.org/fast-fact-330. Accessed on 15 Jan 2019.
9. POLST Care Continuum Toolkit. https://polst.org/wp-content/uploads/2018/01/2018.01.31-POLST-Care-Continuum-Toolkit.pdf. 2018. Accessed on 15 Jan 2019.

Chapter 20
A Threshold Moment, Preserving Patient Dignity, and the Value of a Time-Limited Trial

Pringl Miller

Case Introduction

Mr. James is a 64-year-old man with a history of type II diabetes, hypertension, hyperlipidemia, Crohn's disease, hepatitis C, and end-stage renal disease s/p renal transplant on an immunosuppressive regimen. He presents to the emergency department with complaints of nausea, vomiting, and diarrhea for 2 weeks. He also complains of buttock pain from a wound with foul smelling drainage.

On physical examination, Mr. James is obese, dehydrated, in rapid atrial fibrillation, with altered mental status, and lethargic. His abdomen is mildly tender. He has a tender draining malodorous left gluteal wound with skin necrosis.

Usual Approach

Admit the patient to the ICU with the diagnosis of diabetic ketoacidosis secondary to sepsis from a gluteal necrotizing skin and soft-tissue infection (necSSTI). Initiate an insulin drip, normal saline IV fluid resuscitation, and parenteral broad-spectrum antibiotics. Consult general surgery to evaluate the left gluteal wound. Patient goes to the operating room (OR) multiple times with multiple surgeons for debridement. The third time, the surgeon diagnoses necrotizing fasciitis despite the patient remaining clinically stable. The surgeon tells the family that he is dying and transfers him to the hospice unit for comfort-focused care.

P. Miller (✉)
Departments of Medicine and Surgery, Rush University Medical Center, Chicago, IL, USA

© Springer Nature Switzerland AG 2020 137
K. Aberger, D. Wang (eds.), *Palliative Skills for Frontline Clinicians*,
https://doi.org/10.1007/978-3-030-44414-3_20

Palliative Approach

The patient is admitted to the ICU and your surgical colleagues are consulted. They recommend emergent CT imaging of the affected left gluteal and surrounding area to rule out a deep-soft tissue infection. The CT is negative and urgent operative exploration and debridement of the superficial necSSTI is recommended. Mr. James undergoes aerobic and anaerobic cultures, soft-tissue debridement of a $13 \times 3 \times 3$ cm area, and pulse lavage. A perianal fistula is suspected because of Mr. James preexisting history of Crohn's disease in the context of presenting with a perianal necSSTI, but was not identified in the OR. Mr. James tolerates the procedure well and goes to the PACU in stable condition.

Between POD 1 and 2, Mr. James continues to suffer from diarrhea. *C. difficile* is diagnosed and treated medically. His renal function normalizes and his allograft remains functional. Pan-sensitive *E. coli* grows out of the intraoperative wound cultures, and his antibiotic regimen is adjusted accordingly. Mr. James responds to therapy as evidenced by his daily subjective and objective clinical assessments.

On POD 3, Mr. James returns to the OR for exploration of his wound due to increased purulent drainage and a concern for persistent infection. During this surgery, Mr. James is diagnosed with a nonsurvivable, rapidly progressive necSSTI that extends deep to the sacrum, into the muscle, and adjacent to the rectum. An additional 225 sq. cm of tissue is debrided before the procedure is aborted. Following surgery, Mr. James is returned to the PACU and extubated.

Three days after Mr. James is admitted, he goes into surgery in stable condition without clinical evidence of deterioration. During surgery, he is diagnosed with a nonsurvivable deep necSSTI. This dramatic change in clinical condition represents a threshold moment for Mr. James and his loved ones as well as a pivotal moment for considering alternative care goals.

Box 1 A Threshold Moment

A threshold moment is a point in care when the differing perspectives of the patient, loved ones, and treatment team may come into conflict. In this case, Mr. James' condition is deemed terminal by one provider despite conflicting data and in the absence of multidisciplinary assessment. It is not surprising that Mr. James, his loved-ones, and nonsurgical treatment teams are perplexed by this sudden turn of events.

The surgical attending contacts Mr. James' wife by phone to relay the intraoperative findings and recommends a transition to comfort-focused care and transfer to the hospice inpatient unit (IPU). The surgical attending then contacts the hospitalist and the hospice and palliative medicine on-call attending to arrange transfer to the hospice IPU. Mr. James' family comes to visit the next day to find the patient awake and comfortable. They become confused and request more information.

Box 2 Preserving Patient Dignity

Joan Cassell, an anthropologist who studied the behavior of surgeons, articulated the perceived dilemma at the center of surgical culture and behavior: "It may be the exceptional surgeon who is capable of recognizing and supporting the autonomy of patients, of allowing them to share decision-making, of acknowledging uncertainty in the face of decisions that must be made."

As important as patient autonomy, is the preservation of patient dignity eloquently described by Harvey Chochinov as "kindness, humanity, and respect – the core values of medical professionalism – are too often being overlooked in the time pressured culture of modern health care, ... the A, B, C, and D of dignity conserving care can reinstate them. Attitude, behavior, compassion, and dialogue provide a framework to guide healthcare providers towards maintaining a patient's dignity. For anyone who has the privilege to care for patients, at whatever stage of the human life cycle, the duty to uphold, protect, and restore the dignity of those who seek our care embraces the very essence of medicine."

A conversation proceeds:

Surgical Attending (SA)	"Mr. James, I would like to discuss what we saw in the operating room, would that be okay with you?"
Mr. James (Pt)	"Yes"
SA	"The infection progressed much more than we anticipated. It wasn't possible for us to safely remove all the infected tissue. I am concerned that we may not be able to treat this infection successfully. I am very sorry to share this information with you." (Silence)
Pt	"What are you saying? Am I dying?"
SA	"I am concerned that we may not be able to control this infection. We have several options moving forward. We will hope for the best and prepare for the worst. We can continue our present management and see how you respond during the next few days. It's important to discuss what your preferences would be if the infection makes you so sick that you can no longer participate in a goals-of-care discussion. Because of that possibility, who or with whom would you want to make medical decisions on your behalf? When I take care of people who have serious infections like this, they often require life support. That means being on a breathing machine or receiving medications to maintain a normal blood pressure. Have you ever thought about needing to be on life support? In this situation we would not want to initiate life support unless that was your preference and we thought life support would be beneficial and temporary." (Pause ...)

Pt   "This is all so sudden…I haven't really thought about it. But if you're tell-
          ing me that I might die because of an infection and there are no remaining
          treatment options, I would not want to be put on life support."
SA   "Mr. James, we will continue to provide all the care we can to treat this
          infection but if it looks like your body is not responding and you are dying,
          I would suggest that we do not intervene with life prolonging interventions
          such as CPR. If it's okay with you I would like your medical record to
          reflect that."
Pt   "Alright."
SA   "So to confirm what we've discussed: The medical team would not inter-
          vene if it looked like you were imminently dying and we would let nature
          take its course?"
Pt   "Yes that's correct."
SA   "Before I go, I want to make sure: Is your pain under control? What else
          can I do to help you and your family through this time?"
Pt   "My pain is controlled with the medicines. I can't think of anything else
          right now. My wife and I may have other questions later."
SA   "That's fine. I want to reassure you that we will continue to update you on
          your condition and continue to discuss your goals of care. We want to
          make sure all your questions are answered and that we honor your wishes."
Pt   "Thank you."

Box 3 Principles in Delivering Difficult News

Honor the right of the patient, or his/her surrogate to determine treatment,
including those that may, or may not, prolong life.

Communicate clearly and candidly with patients, their families, and
caregivers.

Identify the primary goals of care from the patient's perspective, and
address how the surgeon's care can achieve them.

Applying the American College of Surgeons "Principles of Palliative Care" and GUIDE [1] Road Map to Breaking Bad News

G: Get Ready

Be certain the news being delivered is accurate and complete. Understand the emotional significance of the news to the patient and their loved ones. Engage them in
the discussion. This may also include members of the patient's treatment team such
as their primary care physician, nurse, chaplain, social worker, and providers who
have developed rapport with the patient. They may be able to offer additional insight
and skill to ease communication and enhance universal understanding and

consensus. Consider what additional support you can offer to the patient and their family when delivering devastating news. Find a time, a quiet place, silence your devices (get temporary coverage if you need to), and sit with presence facing the patient and/or surrogate.

U: Understand What Your Patient Has Heard Before You Disclose

Consider what the trajectory of the patient's condition has been up until now and what plans and goals of care have already been discussed. Acknowledge your place in the scope of the care being provided. Appreciate that this is their starting point; new information will need to be processed and adjusted to. And also take into consideration that the perception of time is skewed for the seriously ill patient and their family, especially in the ICU [2].

Recognize this is a threshold moment in the life of this patient and his/her family and treat it with the sensitivity the situation deserves. The late essayist and former editor of the *New York Times Book Review* wrote, "To the typical physician my *illness is a routine incident in his rounds while for me it's the crisis of my life. I would feel better if I had a doctor who at least perceived this incongruity*" [3].

In the scenario outlined above, understanding the patient's perspective and his stable condition consider transferring the patient back to the ICU for observation. This would allow all treatment teams to assess the patient, further discuss his/her presumed change in condition, and reach consensus about GOC. Additionally, by admitting the possibility that the patient could exceed the prognosis [4] is humbling for the clinician and may build trust with the patient and family during this transition. Finally, it is essential to give the patient and his/her family time to process the critical change in condition and new prognosis before being inundated with a multitude of medical decisions. A hasty acquisition of new treatment directives may seem impatient and uncaring [4].

I: Inform, or Disclose, the News Using a One-Sentence Headline

"I would like to share with you what we saw in the operating room today. Unfortunately there was more infection present than we anticipated and that we could safely remove surgically."

NOT "We saw pus everywhere and could not do anything else."

D: Deepen Your Connection by Responding to Emotions

Allow there to be a silence and wait for the patient and/or family to speak.

"I can see this is not the news you were expecting or hoping to hear. I'm sorry to have to deliver this news."

E: Finally, Equip Your Patient for the Next Steps in Care

"Mr. James I am concerned about the severity of this infection and the effect of the immunosuppression that's required for maintenance of your kidney transplant. Am I correct in thinking you would like us to continue all current treatment options for this infection at this time? Rest assured we will do everything we can to keep you comfortable and treat the infection moving forward. What's going through your mind right now? Would you like to ask any questions? This is a lot to take in and we can definitely talk later."

Case Continued: A Time-Limited Trial

The patient and family request another meeting later in the day. As observed in this case, surgical decision-making eclipsed an approach of shared decision-making. A shared-decision making approach includes patient–family engagement and an effort to collaborate with all integral multispecialty and interdisciplinary care teams including palliative care when indicated. Not engaging with with key stakeholders risks compromising the quality of patient care. A shared-decision-making approach seeks to engage the stakeholders to reach consensus enabling patient concordant care and avoiding confusion, frustration, and dissatisfaction.

Surgical training and culture often fail to emphasize the advantage of collaborating with the entire treatment team in order to attain the optimal patient-centered care plan. This process usually involves a series of discussions to confirm the patient's preferences and negotiation of future treatment and interventions. In this situation when disease-directed therapy is perceived to border on nonbeneficial treatment and prolongation of suffering, implementing a time-limited trial (TLT) can provide the middle ground satisfactory to everyone.

Surgical teams can lose sight of reaching a consensus because of traditional medical hierarchy and surgical culture. Breaking away from the traditional default of solitary surgical decision-making and embracing a collaborative approach to patient care is a paradigm shift for some surgeons.

"Clinicians, patients and families frequently face scenarios in which they must make decisions near the end of life, i.e. whether to initiate major interventions in uncertain circumstances. They do not want to prematurely forgo treatments that might help, but they also many not want to risk indefinite exposure to burdensome treatments. The possibility of a TLT of treatment may provide a way forward" [5–10].

Quill and Holloway describe a TLT in the context of a serious life limiting illness as an agreement between clinicians and the patient to use certain medical therapies over a defined period to see if the patient improves or deteriorates. If the patient improves, disease-directed therapy continues. If the patient deteriorates, the therapies involved in the trial are withdrawn, and treatment is transitioned to comfort-focused care. If there is clinical uncertainty, another TLT could be negotiated.

Mr. James was not given an opportunity to share his goals of care in the usual approach describe above, nor was he given an option to continue disease-directed therapy albeit within the framework of a TLT. If the surgical attending assessed Mr. James to have a nonsurvivable necSSTI, but had engaged in a shared-decision making process instead of a standard surgical-decision making approach, a reasonable middle ground would have been to continue aggressive measures within the framework of a TLT. That way, Mr. James' wishes would have been honored and the treatment teams would have allowed more time for his clinical trajectory to become apparent. Most importantly, Mr. James and his family would have felt supported during this devastating time in their lives.

Giving a patient and their family a fatal prognosis can be a high stakes declaration. Integrating a TLT into the care of a patient presumed to be near the end of life allows time to align with the patient and their family, adjust care to disease progression, alter goals of care, and provide time to plan. Additionally, for the clinician who finds prognostication challenging, unpredictable and stressful, a TLT is an ideal way to lessen this burden and allow more time for the patient's condition to declare itself. A TLT embraces the tincture of time that will reveal the natural course of disease and usually determine the best path forward. In this way, a partnership is formed with the patient and his/her treatment teams in being aligned and committed to a mutually agreed upon plan of care for a predetermined period of time. If at the end of a TLT the patient shows clinical improvement, indicated interventions may continue on an open-ended basis to satisfy new goals of care. Alternatively, if the patient deteriorates, the TLT interventions may no longer be indicated and/or desired. If there is ambiguity, perhaps another TLT meets the needs of all to wait-and-see.

Case Conclusion

After Mr. James returns to the hospital for a TLT of disease-directed therapy for his necSSTI, his condition improves. He is discharged home 6 days later on POD 10 from his original debridement and drainage procedure. He discharges from the hospital with home-based parenteral antibiotics and clinic follow-up with all his consultants. Mr. James does well and continues to respond to treatment with wound care and progressive healing. His allograft remains functional.

Take-Away Points
- *Recognize* threshold moments in the lives of patients and their families.
- *Honor* patient autonomy and dignity by adopting a shared-decision-making approach to goals of care.
- *Engage* the interdisciplinary and multispecialty care teams for a comprehensive patient concordant care plan.
- *Utilize* time-limited trials as an effective way to proceed when faced with uncertainty in the patients' trajectory or their preferences for treatment. A time-limited trial may be necessary for patients and families to adjust, accept, and prepare for an alternative set of care goals.

Acknowledgments Janet Stark, MD, MBA, Sara Scarlet, MD, MPH, and Kimberly Kopecky, MD, MSci for their insight and editorial feedback.

References

1. Vital tips. Accessed https://apps.apple.com/us/app/vitaltalk-tips/id1109433922
2. Robert C. Macauley, ethics in palliative care - a complete guide 2018.
3. Chochinov HM. Dignity and the essence of medicine: the A, B, C, and D of dignity conserving care. BMJ. 2007;335(7612):184–7. https://doi.org/10.1136/bmj.39244.650926.47.
4. Robert C. Macauley, ethics in palliative care - a complete guide 2018.
5. Quill TE, Holloway R. Time-limited trials near the end of life. JAMA. 2011;306(13):1483–4.
6. Khurana P, et al. Internal Medicine Review. 2017;3(8)
7. Scherer JS, Holley JL. The role of time-limited trials in dialysis decision making in critically ill patients. Clin J Am Soc Nephrol. 2016;11(2):344–53. Accessed https://pdfs.semanticscholar.org/b784/cc87cd8901438964ee09e31a5771449f6635.pdf
8. Shrime MG, et al. Time-limited trials of intensive care for critically ill patients with cancer - how long is long enough? JAMA Oncol. 2016;2(1):76–83. https://doi.org/10.1001/jamaoncol.2015.3336.
9. Schenker Y, et al. Discussion of treatment trials in intensive care. J Crit Care. 2013;28(5):862–9.
10. Neuman MD, et al. Using time-limited trials to improve surgical care for frail older adults. Ann Surg. 2015;261(4):639–41. https://doi.org/10.1097/SLA.0000000000000939.

Chapter 21
Between a Rock and a Hard Place: Anticipating Poor Surgical Outcomes While Honoring Patient Autonomy

Calista M. Harbaugh, Christopher P. Scally, Daniel B. Hinshaw, and Pasithorn A. Suwanabol

Case Introduction

A 65-year-old male with Stage IIIB multiple myeloma, severe chronic obstructive pulmonary disease (COPD) substantially limiting any physical activity, and chronic kidney disease (CKD) is admitted to the intensive care unit (ICU) for treatment of recurrent and refractory *C. difficile* infection. Despite maximal intravenous, oral, and rectal antibiotic therapy, the patient develops worsening abdominal distension with possible compromised bowel. You are the general surgeon on call and your team has been consulted. Your assessment of the patient confirms toxic megacolon. As his illness worsens, his renal function deteriorates into oliguria. Vasopressors are initiated, and his oxygen requirement rapidly escalates.

Usual Approach

You confirm the patient has medical decision-making capacity by ensuring that he is able to understand his condition, appreciate the risks and benefits of treatment options, rationalize his decision, and finally, make a consistent choice [1]. Together

C. M. Harbaugh (✉) · P. A. Suwanabol
Department of Surgery, University of Michigan, Ann Arbor, MI, USA
e-mail: calistah@med.umich.edu; pasuwan@med.umich.edu

C. P. Scally
Department of Surgical Oncology, University of Texas M.D. Anderson Cancer Center, Houston, TX, USA
e-mail: cpscally@mdanderson.org

D. B. Hinshaw
Palliative Care Program, University of Michigan Geriatrics Center, Ann Arbor, MI, USA
e-mail: hinshaw@med.umich.edu

© Springer Nature Switzerland AG 2020
K. Aberger, D. Wang (eds.), *Palliative Skills for Frontline Clinicians*,
https://doi.org/10.1007/978-3-030-44414-3_21

with the patient and his only family who are out of state on speaker phone, you discuss goals of care.

Although he communicates with you that he does not want to pursue dialysis in the event of renal failure, this fact does not emerge when the family joins the conversation. The family urges you, "Don't let him die." You say he would survive the surgery, but he may be very sick with a long and difficult recovery. They remain singularly focused on survival, and the patient concedes to the family's wishes. The patient gives consent and you proceed with an open total colectomy with end ileostomy. Post-op, he continues to decline into multiorgan failure, requiring permanent dialysis, tracheostomy, and long-term nursing care. He becomes increasingly depressed and withdrawn with no local family to provide support.

Palliative Approach

You believe that this operation may save this man's life, but worry about the significant morbidity he will have post-op. He is a very high-risk surgical candidate. If he survives, he will likely need dialysis, possibly a tracheostomy and long-term nursing care. Patients and families often assume that the operation will "fix" everything, and the patient will go back to "normal." You have an obligation to discuss possible scenarios with the patient and family to get an understanding of the patient's goals of care. What is acceptable to him as an outcome?

> **Box 21.1 Be Goal-Directed, Not Disease-Directed**
> The patient is an older adult with multiple chronic medical comorbidities in addition to his acute illness. In such cases, a disease-directed care approach may result in overly aggressive treatment and may not address the patient's health priorities. In comparison, a goal-directed care approach places value on the health outcomes that the patient values most, and treatment decisions are made in accordance [2].

Rather than consulting a palliative care specialist, the initial goal-directed care should be managed by the primary clinician, such as the surgeon. This model of primary palliative care delivery is necessary to address the growing shortage of palliative care specialists and reduce fragmentation of care. Primary palliative care delivered by the primary clinician should include basic symptom management and basic discussions regarding prognosis, goals of treatment, suffering, and code status – skills expected of all clinicians [3].

Decisions may involve not only the goals of the patient but also the goals of the family members who may be required to make decisions. Therefore, it is critically important to include the patient, their support, and others who may make surrogate decisions in a family meeting. Meetings should be held in a quiet, comfortable location and pagers or phones silenced [4].

You begin with the preoperative goals of care discussion with the patient and his family. Prior to this hospitalization, the patient had been quite active. Although he became short of breath with walking, he tells the family that his most important priority is to remain living independently. He is concerned that if he required an oxygen tank, he would not be able to manage his daily care. The family is concerned about the distance they live from the patient, that they would be unable to support him in this goal. You find out that the patient has been on dialysis before, at that time it was temporary. He is adamant about not wishing to pursue long-term dialysis because of the toll it took on his quality of life previously. He has not been able to see his mother in several years – she lives out of state – and his fear is that he will never see her again. His family is surprised by how sick he has become over the last few years and voices concern about seeing him again.

You describe your expectations should the patient elect to pursue an operation. Given his serious illness, you anticipate that he will require a total colectomy with permanent ileostomy. Although it is possible his kidneys might again recover after a period of dialysis, it is most likely that he will require long-term dialysis.

You clearly outline the pathways of care. He may proceed with surgery and suffer the possible complications and likely outcomes. You tell him he would require intubation for the surgery, and with his severe COPD, you expect that he will remain intubated for at least several days. While you imagine that he may eventually wean from the oxygen during the hospitalization or inpatient rehabilitation stay, it is more likely that he will permanently require oxygen.

You describe a second option in the event that the above scenario is not acceptable to him. If he is not willing to be more permanently debilitated and participate in long-term dialysis, then the other option is to transition to comfort care. Comfort care, you describe, is an aggressive focus on symptoms to support his body as he goes through the process of dying. You cannot promise he will live long enough to see his family again.

Box 21.2 Which Framework Is the Best?
A number of frameworks exist for guiding goal-directed care conversations, but little evidence exists as to the superiority of any one method. However, they all serve a common mission: to understand patient goals and align treatment decisions with goals. Examples of frameworks include best case/worst case [5], REMAP (reframe, expect emotion, map out patient goals, align with goals, and propose a plan) [6], and SPIKES (setup, perceptions, invitation, knowledge, empathize, summarize, and strategize) [7]. Use the method with which you feel most comfortable eliciting an in-depth understanding of the patient's values with a focus on functional and cognitive outcomes important to the patient's anticipated quality of life. Regardless of framework, effective communication during family meetings should include establishing trust, respect, support, hope, and attention to affect [4]. All relevant persons, including the patient, family members, and health-appointed decision-makers, should be involved in this conversation to provide a roadmap for future treatment decisions.

His family remains focused on survival, failing to appreciate the toll that illness and recovery will take. Although you share with them risk scores for complication rates including death, the family continues to urge you to "try everything." They tell you stories of another family member who required surgery to remove part of his colon and reached full recovery (albeit a middle-aged family member with few medical comorbidities who presented with diverticulitis). The family assures the patient they are coming to be with him and encourages him to fight this. The patient agrees with some obvious misgivings. He says to you – at least with the operation I may live long enough to see them again.

Box 21.3 Your Guidance Demystifies the Potentially Long Journey to Come

Patients and families may not understand the physical and emotional toll associated with undergoing an operation and the relevant risk of adverse outcomes. Stories of others who were surgically cured, and inaccurate media depictions of intense illness and heroic saves, lead to unrealistic expectations [8]. In addition, they neither capture the days, weeks, and months of postoperative recovery nor the residual deficits in quality of life that linger after a major operation.

The preoperative discussion defines the direction of postoperative care and creates an informal contract between surgeon and patient. From the surgeon's perspective, this discussion creates a commitment to the technical aspects of the operation and to the postoperative surgical care and includes shared hope, shared risk, and mutual respect [9]. Postoperative care should be explicitly described (i.e., potential for prolonged life support) in a narrative to place expectations for care into familiar language to the patient and family [10].

Case Continued

You proceed with an uneventful operation; exploratory laparotomy, total abdominal colectomy, and end ileostomy are performed. Postoperatively, the patient is transferred to your service. His hemodynamics rapidly improve and he is extubated within a few days. He continues to require renal replacement therapy without evidence of renal recovery. By now, the entire family including his aging mother has arrived at his bedside.

On postoperative day 5, plans are initiated for transition to intermittent dialysis in anticipation of future discharge to an inpatient rehabilitation facility. However, conflict begins to arise among the patient and his family. The patient is adamant that intermittent dialysis will limit his quality of life and he wishes to cease dialysis. Having seen the patient's recovery thus far, the family is not willing to accept his decision. The patient won't make this decision to pursue comfort care unless his family is in agreement.

Each time you see the patient, he appears increasingly depressed. He will not leave his bed and he speaks very little when his family is present. When his family leaves, he conveys tearful regret for proceeding with surgery and begs you to make his family change their mind. When you try and speak with them, they become increasingly angry and demand a second opinion.

Usual Approach

Unable to reconcile the patient's goals of care with the family's wishes, the case begins to wear on you. The patient is ready to transfer to inpatient rehabilitation on intermittent dialysis, giving you an opportunity to withdraw from the case. You sign the contentious case over to the medical team assuming his care.

Palliative Approach

Rather than transition his care, you approach with a new strategy: You reach out to the specialist palliative care team. The palliative specialist agrees to come to speak with the patient and family to help navigate the difficult situation.

> **Box 21.4 Concurrent Palliative Care Can Augment Surgical Care**
> Consultation for specialist palliative care should be considered for more complex cases. For example, indications for specialist palliative care consultation include need for assistance with conflict resolution regarding goals or treatment methods, management of refractory pain, management of complex mental health symptoms or existential distress, or assistance for addressing cases of near futility [3]. Interprofessional collaboration, particularly in difficult cases, is associated with improvements in the timing and delivery of palliative care [11]. Traditional surgical culture values an aggressive approach, which can be at odds with the patient's values. Integration of palliative care specialists into an interdisciplinary team can aid in elucidation of patient values and promote focus on symptom management, regardless of curative therapeutic intent [12].

Working closely with you, the palliative care physician helps to again navigate goals of care conversations in light of the current situation. The physician aligns the treatment options with the patient's goals of care. The patient and his family finally come together and request to cease dialysis and transition to hospice. Although the family is grieving, the patient and family are all happy that he underwent surgery to allow the patient's family to be at bedside. Ten days later, the patient dies peacefully in hospice with family surrounding him.

Although in line with the patient's goals, you are constantly reminded and bothered by the case. By current 30-day quality metrics, a patient mortality is a failure. Presenting at your department's morbidity and mortality conference, you are met by questions that echo your concerns.

Box 21.5 30-Day Postoperative Mortality: Disincentivizing Best Care
Patient mortality in the postoperative period is often viewed as a failure on the part of the surgeon, regardless of whether care was electively transitioned to comfort care. Furthermore, current measures of quality of care are not centered on patient values and punish surgeons who may already be experiencing their own punishment for unanticipated outcomes. For example, 30-day mortality rates commonly used by hospital ranking and reimbursement systems do not account for transitions to comfort care that respects patient autonomy [13]. For example, when 30-day mortality rate in a trauma ICU was adjusted to exclude comfort care cases not due to failure of therapy, the adjusted mortality rate decreased by 23%. This mortality rate inflation may have negative implications for provider behaviors and reimbursement [14]. Single metrics such as the 30-day mortality rate fail to capture long-term survival, quality of life, and patient-centered outcomes, but currently remain a leading metric for surgical quality reporting and place undue pressure on the surgeon.

Box 21.6 Be Mindful of Second Victim Syndrome
When an adverse event occurs, the provider may also experience emotional and psychological effects collectively called the "second victim syndrome." This is characterized by feelings of failure, followed by a sense of chaos, and finally recovery. Throughout this process, clinical care may be affected and the ability of providers to reflect on events [15, 16]. This process may contribute to burnout. Burnout among surgeons is a pressing and current issue, particularly for younger ones. Training programs have continued to develop and refine surgical education approaches, but wellness initiatives remain a critical gap [17]. It is important that surgeons are equipped with strategies to mitigate the effects of provider burnout, depression, and suicidal ideation.

You reach out to the palliative care team to discuss your difficulty and the questions you are getting from your colleagues regarding the case. The palliative care physician is trained as both a surgeon and a palliative care specialist, allowing her unique insight and perspective. She listens intently and offers you space and presence to process the case emotionally. She acknowledges the pressure placed on you from both internal expectations and external metrics. She also reminds you that your responsibility is to the patient and reassures you that aiding the patient in pursuing hospice is in line with the patient's values and wishes. You leave with a sense of comfort and growth, as well as an enriched sense of what it means for you to be a surgeon.

Traditional surgical metrics would deem this case as a failure – the surgical team was placed accountable for imposing the pain and stress of an operation, then supporting the patient in his decision to cease dialysis. However, it was exactly this approach that allowed the patient to achieve his goals, including time with family and maintaining autonomy, and to die peacefully. With this case, we propose an enhanced model for palliative care in which focus is both on the patient and the invested surgical team. The palliative care physician's role went beyond support of the patient and family, to support of the surgical team. This helped to build stronger networking relationship that will benefit not only this patient but also other patients who might benefit from earlier palliative care involvement in the future.

Take-Away Points
1. The surgeon's role in primary palliative care should consist of basic symptom management and discussions of prognosis, goals of treatment, suffering, and code status.
2. Goal-directed care should be used to align treatment decisions with functional outcomes important to the patient's anticipated quality of life. Several frameworks exist to help guide the discussion to elucidate a patient's health priorities.
3. Specialist palliative care consultation is indicated in the setting of complex symptom management, futile care, and assistance in navigating interpersonal conflict.
4. Quality metrics and the traditional surgeon mentality may be in conflict with goal-directed care. Seeking help for the surgeon to navigate through resistance, frustration, acceptance, and finally healing in difficult cases may lessen the emotional toll of unexpected outcomes.

Disclosure/Conflict of Interest Dr. Amy Suwanabol wishes to disclose research funding from the University of Michigan Division of Geriatric and Palliative Medicine Pilot and Exploratory Award and the Thomas R. Russell Faculty Research Fellowship from the American College of Surgeons. This research received no specific funding/grant from any funding agency in the public, commercial, or not-for-profit sectors. The authors declare no conflicts of interest.

References

1. Leo RJ. Competency and the capacity to make treatment decisions: a primer for primary care physicians. Prim Care Companion J Clin Psychiatry. 1999;1(5):131–41.
2. Tinetti ME, Naik AD, Dodson JA. Moving from disease-centered to patient goals-directed Care for Patients with Multiple Chronic Conditions: patient value-based care. JAMA Cardiol. 2016;1(1):9–10.
3. Quill TE, Abernethy AP. Generalist plus specialist palliative care–creating a more sustainable model. N Engl J Med. 2013;368(13):1173–5.
4. Marks AD, Vitale CA. Caring for patients with limited prognosis: negotiating goals of care and planning for the end-of-life. In: Williams BC, Malani PN, Wesorick DH, editors. Hospitalists' guide to the care of older patients. Hoboken: John Wiley & Sons; 2013. p. 47–64.
5. Taylor LJ, Nabozny MJ, Steffens NM, et al. A framework to improve surgeon communication in high-stakes surgical decisions: best case/worst case. JAMA Surg. 2017;152(6):531–8.
6. Childers JW, Back AL, Tulsky JA, Arnold RM. REMAP: a framework for goals of care conversations. J Oncol Pract. 2017;13(10):e844–50.
7. Baile WF, Buckman R, Lenzi R, Glober G, Beale EA, Kudelka AP. SPIKES-A six-step protocol for delivering bad news: application to the patient with cancer. Oncologist. 2000;5(4):302–11.
8. Serrone RO, Weinberg JA, Goslar PW, et al. Grey's anatomy effect: television portrayal of patients with trauma may cultivate unrealistic patient and family expectations after injury. Trauma Surg Acute Care Open. 2018;3:e000137.
9. Schwarze ML, Bradley CT, Brasel KJ. Surgical "buy-in": the contractual relationship between surgeons and patients that influences decisions regarding life-supporting therapy. Crit Care Med. 2010;38(3):843–8.
10. Pecanac KE, Kehler JM, Brasel KJ, et al. It's big surgery: preoperative expressions of risk, responsibility, and commitment to treatment after high-risk operations. Ann Surg. 2014;259(3):458–63.
11. Khateeb R, Puelle MR, Firn J, Saul D, Chang R, Min L. Interprofessional rounds improve timing of appropriate palliative care consultation on a hospitalist service. Am J Med Qual. 2018;33(6):569–75.
12. Berlin A, Kunac A, Mosenthal AC. Perioperative goal-setting consultations by surgical colleagues: a new model for supporting patients, families, and surgeons in shared decision making. Ann Palliat Med. 2017;6(2):178–82.
13. Schwarze ML, Brasel KJ, Mosenthal AC. Beyond 30-day mortality: aligning surgical quality with outcomes that patients value. JAMA Surg. 2014;149(7):631–2.
14. Weireter LJ, Collins JN, Britt RC, Novosel TJ, Britt LD. Withdrawal of care in a trauma intensive care unit: the impact on mortality rate. Am Surg. 2014;80(8):764–7.
15. Luu S, Patel P, St-Martin L, et al. Waking up the next morning: surgeons' emotional reactions to adverse events. Med Educ. 2012;46(12):1179–88.
16. Marmon LM, Heiss K. Improving surgeon wellness: the second victim syndrome and quality of care. Semin Pediatr Surg. 2015;24(6):315–8.
17. Campbell DA, Sonnad SS, Eckhauser FE, Campbell KK, Greenfield LJ. Burnout among American surgeons. Surgery. 2001;130(4):696–702; discussion 702–695.

Chapter 22
Surgery for the Hospice Patient: When Is It Appropriate?

T. Johelen Carleton

Case Introduction

Mr. Alexander is a 78-year-old male with a long history of metastatic renal carcinoma who was recently diagnosed with a pathologic right femoral fracture.

He resides in a long-term care facility. He is bedbound and in pain despite staggering doses of opioids, including methadone. He is receiving hospice services and is not to be resuscitated. The nursing home staff is distressed over Mr. Alexander's condition. He is clearly frail and looks as if he "wouldn't tolerate a haircut, much less surgery." In fact, prior to your arrival, the nursing home physician and the orthopedic surgeon have considered his risk profile, comorbidities, and functional status, and agreed against operative intervention. You are asked to assist with pain control because the traction dislodges. Not only has his pain increased, but also a sharp spike of femur threatens to puncture his thin skin with little muscle or fat to protect him from an open fracture.

Usual Approach

You accept the decisions that were already made regarding foregoing surgical intervention. You do your best with complex pain control and consider palliative sedation. Unfortunately, the bone punctures the skin and synovial fluid pours out. Wound care implements dressings and suction systems that create more pain especially when they are changed. They are not very effective; the sheets are always wet, his skin is macerated, and he develops pressure ulcers.

T. J. Carleton (✉)
Medical Director Palliative Care, Tucson Medical Center, Tucson, AZ, USA

© Springer Nature Switzerland AG 2020
K. Aberger, D. Wang (eds.), *Palliative Skills for Frontline Clinicians*,
https://doi.org/10.1007/978-3-030-44414-3_22

Palliative Approach

You perform an objective assessment of his operative risk using a validated tool that includes frailty. You prefer the Risk Analysis Index as it has been validated for measuring frailty in surgical populations[2] (Fig. 22.1). The major contributors to his risk are cachexia, poor functional status, and oxygen dependence from pulmonary metastases and COPD. You speak with anesthesia, ICU, and surgery, who all agree that the risk is high, but not prohibitive. As a team, you consider what type of anesthesia would be safest for him. With consensus that repair of the fracture is a viable option and with more objective information about the risks and benefits of surgery, you revisit the goals of care with Mr. Alexander and his medical power of attorney.

Mr. Alexander readily accepts the risks of surgery, including the possibility of death, if it will improve his pain control and quality of life. His medical power of attorney supports his choice. You discuss code status and the rationale for a full resuscitation in the perioperative period. You help Mr. Alexander, his medical power of attorney, the anesthesiologist, the intensivist, and the surgeon, come to a consensus that he will be resuscitated if necessary in the operating room, but revert to an order for no resuscitation immediately afterward.

He is taken to the operating room and the repair is completed in 20 minutes through two small incisions and with minimal hardware. General anesthesia is chosen for the superior physiologic control. Mr. Alexander is extubated in the operating room without difficulty and spends less than 24 hours in the intensive care unit before he transfers back to the nursing home. His opioids are weaned. He is able to get into a wheelchair and visit with friends. He is grateful for the substantial improvement in his quality of life.

Case Continued

Six months later, after a few days of mild constipation, Mr. Alexander develops abdominal discomfort and regrets his decision to participate in the institutionally prepared turkey dinner celebrating the holidays. His abdomen is distended but soft and relatively benign. The plain film shows free air under the right hemidiaphragm.

Usual Approach

Free air is an indication for surgical abdominal exploration. You speak with Mr. Alexander and his medical power of attorney and explain this probably is a critical problem without recourse to intervention. You offer continued hospice or surgery. The do-not-resuscitate order is rescinded, and Mr. Alexander is taken to the operating room. He survives the surgery, but declines rapidly in the following 2 weeks.

Risk Analysis Index (RAI)

Last Name: _____   Last Four: _____

Date From is Completed: _____   Date & Type of Anticipated Surgery:_____

A. Age, Sex & Cancer

Age	Score without Cancer	Score with Cancer
≤ 69	2	20
70–74	3	19
75–79	4	18
80–84	5	17
85–89	6	16
90–94	7	15
95–99	8	14
100+	9	13

1. Sex   Female= 0   Male= 5   _____
2. Age   _____
3. Does the patient have cancer?
   (Excluding skin cancer, except for melanoma)
   If no, score *without* cancer _____
   or
   If yes, score *with* cancer _____

B. Medical Co-Morbidities

4. Have you had unintentional weight loss in the past 3 months (>10 lbs)?   No= 0 Yes= 5 _____
5. Renal failure?   No= 0 Yes= 6 _____
6. Chronic/congestive heart failure?   No= 0 Yes= 4 _____
7. Poor appetite?   No= 0 Yes= 4 _____
8. Shortness of breath (at rest)?   No= 0 Yes= 8 _____

C. Cognition, Residence & Activity of Daily Living

9. Do you reside in a setting other than independent living?
   If yes, check answer: Skilled nursing facility□   Assisted living □   Nursing home □
   No= 0 Yes= 8 _____

   If yes, were you admitted within the past 3 months?   No □ Yes□

D. Activities of Daily Living & Cognitive Decline *(Circle score for each ADL)*

10. Mobility/Locomotion	11. Eating	12. Toilet Use	13. Personal Hygiene
0. Independent	0. Independent	0. Independent	0. Independent
1. Supervised	1. Supervised	1. Supervised	1. Supervised
2. Limited assistance	2. Limited assistance	2. Limited assistance	2. Limited assistance
3. Extensive assistance	3. Extensive assistance	3. Extensive assistance	3. Extensive assistance
4. Total Dependence	4. Total Dependence	4. Total Dependence	4. Total Dependence

14. Have your cognitive skills or status deteriorated over the past 3 months? No □ Yes□ *(see score chart)*

ADL Score without Cognitive Decline *(Sum of ADI Scores)*	ADL Score with Cognitive Decline
0	ADL Score -2
1,2	ADL Score -1
3,4	ADL Score 0
5–7	ADL Score +1
8,9	ADL Score +2
10,11	ADL Score +3
12,13	ADL Score +4
14–16	ADL Score +5

Score *without* cognitive decline _____ (0 to 16)
or
Score *with* cognitive decline _____ (−2 to 21)

Total RAI Score: _____

Fig. 22.1 RAI-C questionnaire and scoring system. Scoring instructions: to calculate the RAI-C score, first look at the Age/Cancer table to determine the single value between 2 and 20 that corresponds to the patient's age and cancer status. Record this single value in the appropriate line for item 3. Next look at the ADL table and sum the scores (0–4) for the four ADLs queried in items 10–13. This sum is the ADL score and should range between 0 and 16. Next look at the ADL/Cognitive-Decline table to determine the single value between −2 and 21 that corresponds to the patient's ADL score and cognitive decline. Record the value in the appropriate line for item 14. Finally, sum the values for items 1, 3–9, and 14 to yield a final RAI-C score between 0 and 81. (© 2016 American Medical Association. All rights reserved.)

Palliative Approach

You speak with Mr. Alexander and his medical power of attorney. You explain that unlike last time, the present risk and the stress of an intra-abdominal exploration, and removal of pathology once detected, are much greater than the straightforward repair of a femoral fracture. You also explain that in some instances, there may be resolution with nonoperative management, but death remains a very real possibility. You ask Mr. Alexander what he thinks about the choice before him. He believes he will not survive surgery. He doesn't want to be in the intensive care unit on mechanical support especially if he's likely to die anyway, and he isn't really feeling that bad. There is a consensus for nonoperative management, understanding the decision may be fatal. Mr. Alexander is willing to be NPO for bowel rest but he does not want a nasogastric tube for decompression, understanding his increased risk of aspiration. The following morning, he insists on coffee. For weeks afterward, he enjoys talking about how one surgery helped him and how avoiding another surgery helped him too. Mr. Alexander lives several more months with what he deems an acceptable quality of life before he dies due to the pulmonary complications of metastatic renal cell carcinoma.

Take-Away Points
1. A patient on hospice still requires discussion of "elective" interventions, even invasive surgery, especially if they may palliate symptoms.
2. Objective frailty and functional status measures are important predictors of surgical outcomes and overall prognosis. The Risk Analysis Index 2 is one method to evaluate your patient.
3. A surgical emergency in a frail and declining patient does not necessarily require surgery if it will not add to the patient's quality of life or overall survival.
4. Patient-centered surgical decisions in the frail and elderly require complex, coordinated communication among multiple disciplines.
5. Good surgical care is good palliative care.

Suggested Reading

1. Kwok AC, Semel ME, Lipsitz SR, Bader AM, Barnato AE, Gawande AA, Jha AK. The intensity and variation of surgical care at the end of life: a retrospective cohort study. Lancet. 2011;378(9800):1408–13. https://doi.org/10.1016/S0140-6736(11)61268-3.
2. Ernst KF, Hall DE, Schmid KK, Seever G, Lavedan P, Lynch TG, Johanning JM. Surgical palliative care consultations over time in relationship to systemwide frailty screening. JAMA Surg. 2014;149(11):1121–6. https://doi.org/10.1001/jamasurg.2014.1393.

3. Hall DE, Arya S, Schmid KK, Blaser C, Carlson MA, Bailey TL, Purviance G, Bockman T, Lynch TG, Johanning J. Development and initial validation of the risk analysis index for measuring frailty in surgical populations. JAMA Surg. 2017;152(2):175–82. https://doi.org/10.1001/jamasurg.2016.4202.
4. Schwarze ML, Bradley CT, Brasel KJ. Surgical "buy-in": the contractual relationship between surgeons and patients that influences decisions regarding life-supporting therapy. Crit Care Med. 2010;38(3):843–8. https://doi.org/10.1097/CCM.0b013e3181cc466b.

Chapter 23
Nonoperative Approach to Caring for the Ischemic Limb

Rachel Danczyk and Erika Ketteler

Case Introduction

A 92-year-old man is brought to the Veteran's Affairs (VA) emergency department by his fiancée and family friend. He has had multiple falls the last few days, worsening mental status in the setting of dementia, and anorexia. Per his fiancée, he seems to be favoring his left leg. During evaluation in the ED, he is noted to have a cool left lower extremity with mottling and absent pulses. His fiancée states that she is in the middle of transferring his care from a community hospital to the VA.

The patient is unable to give any recent history but appears to be comfortable lying in bed. His left leg is pulseless, cold, and mottled. His right leg appears normal and has palpable pulses at the foot and behind the knee.

Usual Approach

You discuss with his fiancée and friend that his left leg has no blood flow and needs emergent surgery to restore blood flow for best pain control and outcome. You then take him to the OR and perform exploration of the left femoral artery with thromboembolectomy, arteriography, and possible revascularization with endovascular or open bypass procedures, and fasciotomies of the left calf. He returns to the surgical ICU after surgery, is intubated, and is closely monitored and resuscitated.

R. Danczyk
University of New Mexico Department of Surgery, Albuquerque VA Medical Center, Albuquerque, NM, USA

E. Ketteler (✉)
Raymond G. Murphy VAMC, Albuquerque, NM, USA
e-mail: Erika.Ketteler@va.gov

© Springer Nature Switzerland AG 2020
K. Aberger, D. Wang (eds.), *Palliative Skills for Frontline Clinicians*,
https://doi.org/10.1007/978-3-030-44414-3_23

His DNAR order is suspended for the time in surgery and for a minimum 48 hours post surgery. His postoperative pain and delirium are difficult to manage. He has a prolonged ICU stay, and finally stabilizes to transfer to the floor where he fails a swallow evaluation. A feeding tube is placed and the patient is sent to a subacute rehab facility. He is readmitted 3 days later with pneumonia, codes in the ICU, and dies an hour later.

Palliative Approach

While evaluating the patient, his fiancée says he recently underwent hip replacement and is using a walker for assistance. She quickly states that she is worried about him returning home since her family friends are going out of town in the next few days and will not return for several weeks. She also states that the patient recently "graduated" hospice for congestive heart failure and was doing well at home prior to the last few days. When asked about his care at home, the fiancée is notably upset and says he was doing better in her care than with home hospice.

Box 23.1 Doing More by Doing Less
You have some reconciling to do. Surgeons are trained to operate and use technical skills to cure or alleviate pain. Historically the "simplest" way to take care of a patient such as described in this case was to convince the patient and family that an operation is the only way to treat the acute situation and control the pain. This "doing" rather than "listening" seems so much easier and feels like it takes much less time. However, such an approach is not shared decision-making and not acting in the role as surgeon advocate for your patient. To listen and assess what the patient and family goals are really doesn't take much time, and consequently, decision-making is truly shared.

Most surgeons feel comfortable offering a solution that is in line with how they were trained to DO rather than exploring other options of LISTENING. This shift in approach at first may seem unpalatable, but ultimately is fully in line with best surgical care that evaluates risks, benefits, and alternatives that are consistent with patient and family goals and wishes. By becoming familiar, and more importantly comfortable, with using conversation as a surgical instrument, good palliative care is good surgical care.

After his fiancée mentions her fears regarding taking him home and not being able to care for him alone, you pause and take some time to discuss her understanding of his illnesses, prognosis of his current diagnoses, and what the patient would want done in an emergency if he could speak for himself. You seek to discern whether the patient would agree to this surgery in an emergency, and what the patient and his fiancée's greatest fears are now.

She tells you that she knows he is dying from his dementia and heart failure and that his leg is hurting him. She states that although she is scared of losing him, she knows he would not want surgery, even to save his life or limbs. More than anything else, she fears he is in pain. She expresses that they both have an understanding that he should not have surgery, remain DNAR, and focus medical efforts on keeping him comfortable. She states that she would like him to stay in the hospital to keep him pain free, but knows this conflicts with his desire to die at home.

Box 23.2 Amputation May Not Always Be the Answer

When treating frail patients who are near dying with an ischemic limb, some surgeons may hesitate and offer amputation even though it is well known that amputation does not always lead to less pain and suffering for the patient. For most surgeons who would opt to amputate, their decision does not reflect their ignorance or their unwillingness to listen to the patient's wishes. Rather, many may feel burdened with the thought of an odorous and unsightly leg becoming the centerpiece of a patient's last days. You may worry that you will be burdened with leaving your patient with a nonviable leg. You envision a horrific picture of a patient in pain, leaving family to negotiate with hospice care or even return to the emergency department.

With the help of your palliative care colleagues at your institution, you now understand that there are very specific strategies to truly palliate the patient with an ischemic limb that does not necessarily have to include surgery, especially for a patient who is actively dying on presentation.

Together with the patient's family and friends, you decide to admit the patient to your surgical inpatient service for acute hospice care. You have created a trusting relationship with the family and understand the goal of the medical care for the immediate time frame. Your team focuses on the patient's pain, so it can be managed initially with IV medications until a home hospice care transition can occur. With the help of the consulting palliative care team, you work to see if home care is an option.

There are useful and validated approaches from the palliative care literature that you utilize in this patient to care for an ischemic leg that does not require surgery. You educate the family on the use of dark stockings or wound boots to mask the discoloration, betadine paint to treat open wounds and control odor at the surface, and ground coffee or cat litter in the room to further mask odor.

> **Box 23.3 Better Together**
> By spending some time with the palliative care team either on rounds or in a multidisciplinary team setting of your choice, you can gain invaluable information and strategies to enhance your current surgical palliative care skills. More importantly, by partnering with other surgeons interested in palliative approaches to surgical care, you will feel empowered to make decisions based on your patient's values. Fostering support for surgeons in your facility who choose nonoperative care pathways consistent with patient and family goals is critical to providing patient-centered medical and surgical care.

You discuss with the family that every effort will be made to minimize interruptions and that vital signs will not be checked and no neurovascular exams will be performed. The team will focus on pain control and comfort and allow access to foods from home if the patient prefers. Visitors will not be limited. Chaplain service will be notified. Social work will assist in measures of returning to care at home. Delirium will be recognized and appropriate comfort measures instituted proactively. You, as the surgeon, focus on all aspects of the patient and his fiancée's suffering: the physical, the spiritual, the social, and the psychological. Given the patient's dementia, concern is raised by nursing as to how best identify and treat his pain. The patient with severe dementia can accurately be evaluated as experiencing pain and treated with good control that is consistent with quality palliative care.

> **Box 23.4 Better Together**
> Bedside assessment of pain in patients with nonverbal dementia focuses on key elements of the patient's behavior rather than their verbal expressions:
>
> - Facial expressions
> - Vocalizations
> - Body movements
> - Changes in interpersonal interactions
> - Changes in patterns or routines
> - Mental status changes

With careful assessments and coordination with the nursing team, you successfully manage his symptoms nonoperatively rather than through the conventional surgical approach. The patient is kept comfortable; however, his delirium and agitation worsen, and unfortunately, returning home is no longer an option. With your palliative care team's assistance, he is started on scheduled medications and becomes more comfortable and somnolent. Later that day, the patient dies with his fiancée at his side. The family is grateful for a peaceful death and is thankful he did not suffer or have to undergo an operation in his last days of life.

You are grateful that you listened to your inner voice of total patient care rather than your inner voice of surgical dogma. Surgeons have great potential (and have natural expertise!) to become the best listeners and advocates for patients if they remain open to using all the instruments they have available to them. This includes being familiar with stressful and urgent crises where listening, reason, and calm, clear communication are beneficial rather than innuendos or avoidance. You vow to continue to look for the best options available when it comes to providing care for your patients, not just the option in which you are most familiar.

Take-Away Points
1. Listen to your patient and their family to get the best sense of their wishes; ask rather than tell.
2. Probe the hard questions regarding amputation risks and benefits in the setting of limb ischemia; use best case/worst case discussions.
3. Know your nonoperative alternatives when taking care of a patient with limb ischemia.
4. Invest in learning from palliative care specialists to improve surgeon skills in communication and managing symptoms at the end of life.

Chapter 24
Placing a Feeding Tube in a Patient with Dementia

Jay A. Requarth

Case Introduction

Mrs. R is an 89-year-old woman with Alzheimer's dementia. She is recently widowed by her husband of 50 years whom she cared for throughout the course of his dementia and death. After his death, she declined, needing full-time care and was admitted to a nursing home. She had a recent hospitalization for a femur fracture complicated by an infected decubitus ulcer. In order to receive antibiotics, the family decided to place a feeding tube. The patient is now admitted with aspiration pneumonia despite the feeding tube. There have been numerous complications with the tube, including leakage and the patient pulling it out repeatedly. At this time, the chronic leakage around the tube has caused associated painful skin burns. The family is requesting that the feeding tube be removed. The nursing home has notified adult protective services as they feel the family is "starving" the patient.

Usual Approach

You treat the aspiration pneumonia, place a larger tube, and send the patient back to the nursing facility to sort out the details of the patient's care and feeding.

The family will go against the nursing home administration and adult protective services, but the feeding tube is maintained. Mrs. R is agitated and pulls at her tubes. She ends up restrained and sedated, laying in her own stool. She is admitted multiple times with continuous overall decline, and finally codes on one of her admissions to the hospital for feeding tube-related complications.

J. A. Requarth (✉)
Wake Forest School of Medicine, Winston Salem, NC, USA

© Springer Nature Switzerland AG 2020　　　　　　　　　　　　　　　　165
K. Aberger, D. Wang (eds.), *Palliative Skills for Frontline Clinicians*,
https://doi.org/10.1007/978-3-030-44414-3_24

Box 24.1 The Momentum Toward Artificial Nutrition
Families are very reluctant to allow their loved ones to "starve to death" even when the patient is already not eating because they have lost the will or ability to eat. Furthermore, many nursing homes are reluctant to accept a dementia patient without a feeding tube because the nursing cost associated with careful hand-feeding is just too high. Thus, feeding tubes are commonly placed in the elderly for dysphagia, esophageal dysmotility, or dysphagia associated with dementia. Feeding tubes are placed in 0.8% of Caucasian and 1.7% of African-American Medicare beneficiaries 85 years or older with a 30-day, 1-year, and 3-year survival of 76%, 37%, and 19%, respectively [2].

Palliative Approach

You schedule a family meeting to discuss this matter in detail. Prior to the meeting, you assess how far Mrs. R's dementia has progressed. You see that she has been bed bound since her hip fracture a couple months ago. She can no longer feed herself, is incontinent, and speaks only incoherent words. She does light up when her family comes to visit. She is a Functional Assessment Staging Test (FAST) level 7c [1] (Table 24.1).

Feeding tubes are the classic palliative care procedure. There are three usual reasons for placing a feeding tube: (1) artificial nutrition and hydration (ANH) for dementia, (2) ANH for esophageal and/or gastric dysmotility, and (3) decompression for bowel obstruction. ANH for dementia is not recommended by professional societies, but often requested by families. A surgeon with palliative care communication skills should be able to communicate this paradoxical information to families who want to show their love by saving their family member from starvation.

Box 24.2 Society Guidelines Discourage Artificial Nutrition and Hydration
The Alzheimer's Association, American Geriatrics Society, and American Academy of Hospice and Palliative Medicine recommend against artificial nutrition and hydration in advanced dementia. Careful hand-feeding is encouraged instead, which retains taste of food, socialization, and caregiving.

Although short-term G-tube insertion complications do not differ significantly between patients with and without cognitive disorders [3, 4], a prospective study found no difference in the median 6-month survival of dementia patients in the postfeeding tube group (195 days) versus the nonfeeding tube group (189 days) [5]. Furthermore, Franzoni and colleagues found that carefully supervised hand-feeding is at least as good as tube feeding and may be better for demented patients because it increases

Table 24.1 Functional Assessment Staging Tool for Alzheimer's dementia

Stage	Stage name	Characteristic	Expected untreated AD duration (months)	Mental age (years)	MMSE (score)
1	Normal aging	No deficits whatsoever	–	Adult	29–30
2	Possible mild cognitive impairment	Subjective functional deficit	–		28–29
3	Mild cognitive impairment	Objective functional deficit interferes with a person's most complex tasks	84	12+	24–28
4	Mild dementia	IADLs become affected, such as bill paying, cooking, cleaning, traveling	24	8-12	19–20
5	Moderate dementia	Needs help selecting proper attire	18	5-7	15
6a	Moderately severe dementia	Needs help putting on clothes	4.8	5	9
6b	Moderately severe dementia	Needs help bathing	4.8	4	8
6c	Moderately severe dementia	Needs help toileting	4.8	4	5
6d	Moderately severe dementia	Urinary incontinence	3.6	3–4	3
6e	Moderately severe dementia	Fecal incontinence	9.6	2–3	1
7a	Severe dementia	Speaks 5–6 words during day	12	1.25	0
7b	Severe dementia	Speaks only 1 word clearly	18	1	0
7c	Severe dementia	Can no longer walk	12	1	0
7d	Severe dementia	Can no longer sit up	12	0 5–0.8	0
7e	Severe dementia	Can no longer smile	18	0.2–0.4	0
7f	Severe dementia	Can no longer hold up head	12+	0–0.2	0

person-to-person contact [6]. Thus, there are no data supporting G-tube insertion for dementia patients (FAST level 6–7) who have lost the will or ability to eat [1].

Over the last 50 or so years, medical paternalism has given way to shared decision-making [7]. This was codified with the Patient Self-Determination Act of 1990, which established as US law that a patient's (or surrogate's) right of self-determination is the highest standard of medical ethics [8]. Thus, a patient and/or their surrogate can refuse any medical therapy even if it might prolong their life. However, not providing artificial nutrition and hydration (ANH) requires special consideration in some states; in the other states, the medical power of attorney can unilaterally decide to withhold ANH [9].

Obviously, not providing ANH from a loved one will have immense religious burdens [10]. Pope John Paul II in his 2004 address to the International Conference on Life-Sustaining Treatments and Vegetative State: Scientific Advances and Ethical Dilemmas emphasized the "the administration of water and food, even when provided by artificial means, always represents a *natural means* of preserving life, not a medical act." Thus, according to the Catholic Church, ANH should always be provided to relatively young people in persistent vegetative states where life expectancy is basically limitless. However, ethical and religious directive #58 from the 2009 United States Conference of Catholic Bishops states that providing ANH becomes morally ambiguous when the ANH is not expected to prolong life in patients who are expected to die in the near future.

Case Conclusion

You meet with the family to discuss goals of care. The family is very clear that they believe their mother is suffering and want to allow a natural death without artificial feeding. They request the tube be removed for her comfort to prevent further complications. Based on her clinical condition, her FAST score and her family's goals, it makes sense to transition the patient to comfort care. The family agrees to hospice and the feeding tube is removed.

Take-Away Points
1. Feeding tubes are often placed without intensive discussion with family about realistic goals of care.
2. Surgeons can have goals-of-care discussions based on their own recommendations for placing the tube, despite other doctors advocating placement.
3. There is clear evidence in end-stage dementia that feeding tubes increase the risk of restraint usage, do not prolong life, and do not decrease the risk of aspiration.
4. The bishops of the US Catholic Church do not feel that people need to continue ANH in demented followers of the faith who are near end of life.

References

1. Functional Assessment Staging of Alzheimer's Disease (FAST) scale for dementia. Available at https://www.compassus.com/sparkle-assets/documents/functional-assessment-staging-fast. pdf. Assessed 31 Jan 2019.
2. Grant MD, Rudberg MA, Brody JA. Gastrostomy placement and mortality among hospitalized Medicare beneficiaries. JAMA. 1998;279:1973–6.
3. Van Bruchem-Visser RL, Mattice-Raso FUS, de Beaufort ID, Kulpers EJ. Percutaneous endoscopic gastrostomy in older patients with and without dementia: survival and ethical considerations. J Gastroenterol Hepatol. 2018; [Epub ahead of print].

 4. Clayton S, DeClue C, Lewis T, et al. Radiologic versus endoscopic placement of gastros-
    tomy tube: comparison of indications and outcomes at a tertiary referral center. South Med
    J. 2019;112:39–44.
 5. Gillick M. When the nursing home resident with advanced dementia stops eating: what is the
    medical director to do? J Am Med Dir Assoc. 2001;2:259–63.
 6. Franzoni S, Frisoni GB, Boffelli S, et al. Good nutritional oral intake is associated with equal
    survival in demented and nondemented very old patients. J Am Geriatr Soc. 1996;44:1366–70.
 7. Annas GJ. Informed consent, cancer, and truth in prognosis. N Engl J Med. 1994;330:223–5.
 8. Omnibus Budget Reconciliation Act of 1990, HR 5835, 101st Cong (1990).
 9. Cruzan v Director, Missouri Department of Health, 497 US 261 (1990).
10. United States Conference of Catholic Bishops. Ethical and religious directives for Catholic
    health care services. 5th ed. Available at: http://usccb.org/issues-and-action/human-life-and-
    dignity/health-care/upload/Ethical-Religious-Directives-Catholic-Health-Care-Services-fifth-
    edition-2009.pdf. Updated 17 Nov 2009. Accessed 31 Jan 2019.

Chapter 25
Bowel Obstruction in a Dying Patient: To Operate or Not?

Ana Berlin

Case Introduction

Dora, an 89-year-old woman with end-stage renal disease on peritoneal dialysis (PD), elects to discontinue PD because it no longer meets her goals. She suffers from increasingly frequent bouts of peritonitis requiring repeated hospitalization, as well as fatigue and generalized decline. She tried hemodialysis previously and found it intolerable. Based on the fact that she is not anuric, her prognosis without dialysis is estimated at several weeks.

Dora's goal is to die peacefully of renal failure at home. At her insistence, she is admitted to the surgical service for PD catheter removal, which is uncomplicated. She does well postoperatively and quickly returns to her baseline functional status in the hospital. She is referred for home hospice as was planned preoperatively. When getting out of bed on the morning of her expected discharge home, she feels a sudden "pop" and experiences acute right groin pain. Physical exam reveals a subtle bulge in the right inguinal region and a clinical diagnosis of acutely incarcerated right inguinal hernia is confirmed. Attempts at manual reduction are not successful.

Usual Approach

The surgical team approaches Dora with an offer for emergent inguinal hernia repair with diagnostic laparoscopy and possible bowel resection under general anesthesia. She responds by expressing her wish to avoid interventions and procedures. Based

A. Berlin (✉)
Surgery (Acute Care Surgery) and Medicine (Adult Palliative Medicine), Columbia University Irving Medical Center, New York, NY, USA

© Springer Nature Switzerland AG 2020
K. Aberger, D. Wang (eds.), *Palliative Skills for Frontline Clinicians*,
https://doi.org/10.1007/978-3-030-44414-3_25

on this, and her do not resuscitate (DNR)/do not intubate (DNI) status, the surgical team recommends comfort-focused care.

> **Box 25.1 How should the surgical team respond to patients experiencing acute surgical emergencies near the end of life when they voice their wish to avoid surgical interventions?**
> Most patients prefer to avoid surgical interventions; in a few cases do patients truly "want" surgery. When faced with a patient who declines intervention, a best practice is to explore the rationale for that preference, and the fears, hopes, and values underlying that decision. Patients must understand and accept the consequences of not intervening. In this case, ongoing pain and worsening nausea and vomiting would be expected consequences of a nonoperative approach and are in direct conflict with the patient's expressed goals.
> See Table 25.1 and Fig. 25.1 for two frameworks helpful for communication and decision-making in the emergency surgical setting.
> *Key point: Focus on goals and values, not treatment preferences.*

Table 25.1 A structured framework for acute surgical communication and decision-making with suggested sample phrases (adapted from Cooper et al., *Ann Surg* 2016) [1]

Key step	Specific aims	Sample phrases
Assess prognosis	Assess patient's expected health trajectory and prognosis	*Preparation prior to conversation with patient/surrogate*
Connect and explore	Identify surrogates, express concern for patient's well-being, address symptoms, review prior advance directives, elicit patient/surrogate understanding of health trajectory and prognosis	"Who are the important people in your life? Would you like any of them here with you before we begin talking?" "To be sure we are starting on the same page, can you tell me about her health over the past few months, how things have changed recently, and the problem she is facing today?" "How has your body been treating you lately?" "What has it been like to walk in your shoes?"
Inform	Convey information about the patient's acute problem in the context of the overall health trajectory and expected prognosis	"I'm worried that today's turn of events really changes the course of things…" "I'm afraid the antibiotics have not worked, and the infection has spread."
Summarize	Establish shared understanding: Headline	"What it boils down to is that you've got this new life-threatening crisis on top of an already serious ongoing problem."

Table 25.1 (continued)

Key step	Specific aims	Sample phrases
Pause and empathize	Allow patient/surrogate to process information and express emotion; respond with validation and empathy	"I can see this is really upsetting, and understandably so." "I cannot imagine how hard it is to hear this now." "I am so impressed with the love and dedication you have shown for your sister through all of this."
Describe options	Describe the benefits, burdens, and likely outcomes of available and medically appropriate surgical and nonsurgical options, including palliative treatments	"There are a few different approaches we can take for your problem. Let me tell you what each option might look like for you, in the best case, worst case, and most likely case." "Best case, you would need to recover in a nursing home for a month or two. However, I do think it is quite likely you will not be able to breathe on your own without the ventilator again, in which case you might never be strong enough to make it home."
Elicit and understand goals and values	Understand the patient's goals, values, priorities, acceptable trade-offs, concerns, and limitations; discuss existing advance directives with patient/ surrogate	"Have you ever given any thought to what would be most important for you if you were to get very sick?" "How much are you willing to go through in order to get through this crisis?" "Is there any condition or state you can imagine living in that would be worse than death?"
Recommend	Recommend a course of treatment consistent with the patient's goals; if appropriate, consider a trial of full surgical critical care defined by a clear time frame and parameters for reassessment	"Based on his priorities, I recommend we go to the operating room and do what we can to alleviate your dad's symptoms there. Let's see how things go and plan to meet again in the next 48 hours. If by the end of the week things don't turn around, we should discuss a plan focused on supporting what he has told us is most important to him."
Support	Affirm relationship, summarize next steps to patient/family, document the conversation in the medical record, and communicate the plan to the interdisciplinary team	"We are all committed to providing the best possible care for your wife, and to respecting her goals and priorities." "We will do everything possible that will help with what you've told me matters most to you."

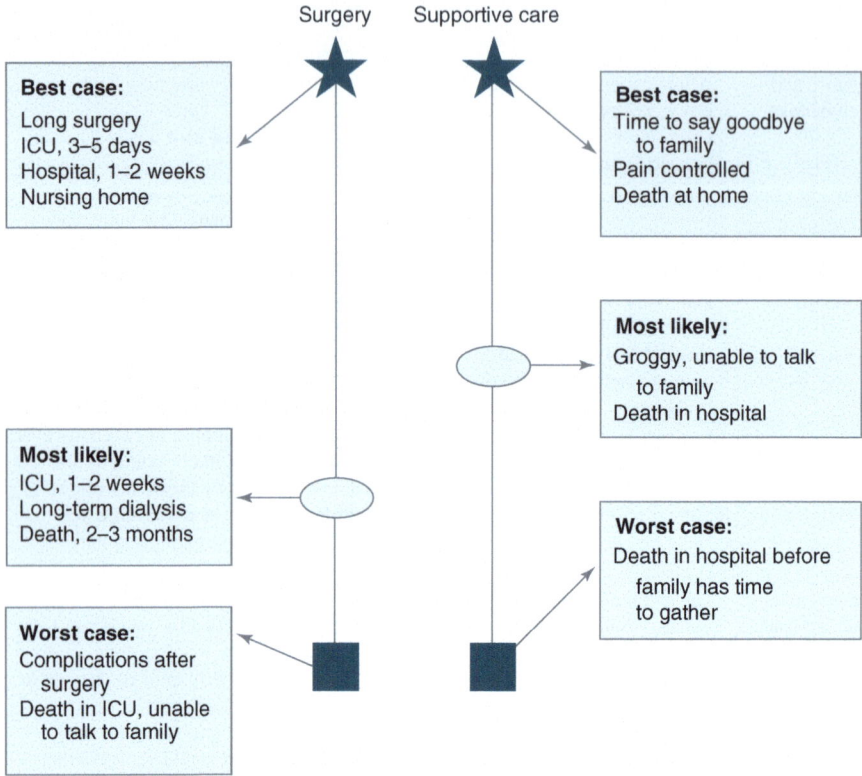

Fig. 25.1 Best-case/worst-case graphic aid. Example of a best-case/worst-case graphic communication aid. The surgeon draws this graphic in real time, so that it serves as the framework for a narrative decision-making conversation with a seriously ill patient/surrogate facing an acute surgical problem. The bars indicate the range of scenarios for the proposed treatment options, the boxes represent the worst-case outcomes, the stars represent the best-case outcomes, and the ovals indicate the most likely outcomes for each option. ICU = intensive care unit [2]. Reproduced with permission from Taylor et al. [2]. Copyright©2017 American Medical Association. All rights reserved

Palliative Approach

Alternatively, the surgical team might consider offering Dora an emergent inguinal hernia repair under local anesthesia. She may likely respond as before, with her wish to avoid interventions and procedures. An exploration of the rationale for these preferences and her underlying goals and values would reveal Dora's fear of pain and discomfort associated with unwanted interventions, as well as her desire to live out her final days in the peace and tranquility of her home. The team might also offer Dora reassurance that the procedure could be performed without revoking her DNR/DNI status.

> **Box 25.2 How should do not resuscitate and do not intubate orders be handled perioperatively?**
> Most hospitals and medical centers now have policies and procedures requiring reconsideration, *not revocation,* of do not resuscitate and do not reintubate orders preoperatively. Such "required reconsideration" policies are in accordance with surgical, anesthesiology, and perioperative nursing professional society recommendations that operating teams caring for patients with established advance directives (including code status limitations) should preoperatively review, discuss, and document specific plans for maintaining, rescinding, or suspending and reinstating these orders in the intraoperative and postoperative periods [3]. These decisions should be made jointly based on consensus among the patient/surrogate, surgeon, anesthesiologist, and operating room nursing staff.
> *Key point: Ensure that advance directives and code status limitations are reviewed, discussed, documented perioperatively, not automatically rescinded.*

With an appropriate invitation from Dora, the surgical team then share a narrative account of the best case, worst case, and most likely scenarios following surgical intervention, as well as alternately describing the worsening symptom burden, accelerated decline, and early death that would be near certain in the event of a nonoperative approach [2]. Based on the discordance between the expected outcome and the Dora's stated goals, the team make a clear recommendation for surgical intervention. Furthermore, by establishing contingency plans for unexpected findings in the operating room or complications postoperatively (e.g., intestinal ischemia requiring resection, inability to tolerate the procedure under local anesthesia with provisions for a time-limited intubation under those circumstances, and clear limitations on intensity of postoperative treatment), Dora feels comfortable proceeding with a relatively low-burden surgical intervention with the goal of palliating her symptoms and allowing her to resume her anticipated and desired end-of-life trajectory. See Table 25.1 and Fig. 25.1 for two frameworks helpful for communication and decision-making in the emergency surgical setting.

Case Continued

Usual Approach

Given her renal failure and highly symptomatic strangulated inguinal hernia, Dora is referred to inpatient hospice for general inpatient level hospice care. By the following day, Dora's groin pain continues to worsen and obstructive symptoms began to manifest in the form of nausea, constipation, and abdominal distension and discomfort. The hernia remains irreducible and evolves to presumed strangulation. Because of difficulty managing her symptoms, the surgical team requests specialty palliative care consultation. Upon evaluation by the palliative care team, Dora understands and expresses resolute acceptance of her shortened prognosis, along with wishes for "comfort" and "no pain or vomiting" and to return home to die peacefully of her renal failure.

The palliative care team establishes trust and rapport with Dora and her family and is able to gently share the news that the patient's goal of returning home would likely not be possible based on the presence of symptoms requiring inpatient management. Given her renal failure and highly symptomatic strangulated inguinal hernia, Dora is referred to inpatient hospice for general inpatient level hospice care. She is assured that every effort will be made to fulfill her wishes for relief of pain and other symptoms. She is accepting and at peace. She is advised that a nasogastric tube for gastrointestinal decompression will likely be necessary to prevent or control the anticipated vomiting that will accompany her incarcerated hernia. She elects to defer until her symptoms worsen. In the meantime, maximal medical antiemetic therapy is scheduled.

Box 25.3 What are the options for maximal medical management of nausea and vomiting associated with intractable benign or bowel obstruction?

The following interventions should be considered and implemented in stepwise fashion:

- Serotonin receptor antagonists ("-setrons") for antiemetic effect at intestinal nausea receptors and cerebral vomiting center
- Dopamine receptor antagonists (e.g., haloperidol 1 mg IV q8h, prochlorperazine 10 mg IV q6h) for antiemetic effect at central receptors
- Prokinetic agents (e.g., metoclopramide 10 mg IV q6h); *only suitable for partial obstruction*
- Anticholinergics (e.g., glycopyrrolate) to decrease bowel secretions and pain from intestinal spasm
- H2 blockers to reduce gastric secretions
- Somatostatin analogs (octreotide) to decrease intestinal secretions and peristalsis
- Corticosteroids (e.g., dexamethasone 4 mg IV q8AM and 2 PM) to decrease bowel edema
- Neurokinin-1 receptor antagonists ("-prepitants") for antiemetic effect at cerebral vomiting center
- Benzodiazepines
- Enteral decompression (nasogastric tube, tube pharyngostomy, venting gastrostomy)

Over the next few days, Dora's pain and gastrointestinal symptoms require escalating therapeutic interventions including scheduled and as-needed opioids, benzodiazepines, and nasogastric decompression. While she is initially able to engage with family and volunteers in narrative life review and legacy-generating activities, she becomes rapidly incapacitated and soon develops hypoactive delirium. Her family remains at her bedside and at peace with her transition. Six days after initially developing her acutely incarcerated hernia, Dora dies comfortably in the hospital.

Palliative Approach

Alternatively, in consultation with her family and surrogate decision-makers, Dora opts to undergo inguinal hernia repair under local anesthesia with the goal of relieving the pain and obstructive symptoms. The surgeon, anesthesiologist, and operating room team all agree with Dora and her surrogates that her DNR order will remain in effect. Her DNI order will be temporarily suspended in the operating room to allow for intubation and general anesthesia, if necessary to comfortably complete the case, with plans to extubate her in the operating room and reinstate the DNI order on arrival to the recovery room. In addition, provisions are put in place for postoperative comfort-focused measures, including palliative extubation while surrounded by family in the event of inability to safely extubate in the operating room. These detailed conversations are carefully documented in the electronic medical record.

In the best-case scenario, Dora receives an open inguinal hernia repair under local anesthesia without a need for bowel resection or intubation. A tension-free repair, using mesh if necessary, would offer Dora the greatest comfort postoperatively, even if recurrence was not a consideration due to her limited life expectancy. Her bowel function returns and electrolytes and fluid balance remain stable despite her renal failure, for long enough to permit discharge home with hospice on postoperative day 1. Her end-of-life trajectory resumes essentially with little change from her baseline status, with an expected prognosis of several weeks.

In the most likely scenario, Dora requires a limited bowel resection for her strangulated hernia, which is completed through the inguinal incision, and a primary hernia repair without mesh. A postoperative ileus requires her to remain in the hospital for another 3 days with enteral decompression before discharge home with hospice as originally planned. Given the fluid shifts associated with a more serious operation and complex postoperative course, once home, she is more debilitated, and on an accelerated decline trajectory. She has a shorter time at home, likely on the order of days, but her end-of-life wishes are realized.

In the worst-case scenario, Dora requires a bowel resection through an extended incision requiring intubation in the operating room. Despite postoperative extubation and comfort-focused care, her course is complicated by intraabdominal sepsis due to anastomotic breakdown requiring intravenous analgesia and sedation. She has a rapid descent into hypoactive delirium and death in the hospital on general inpatient level hospice care within several days of the operation.

Case Conclusion

This case illustrates how palliative care principles can and should be integrated concurrently with the best surgical care. For patients with acute reversible surgical problems in the course of an otherwise subacute terminal illness, operative intervention can be central to a palliative strategy of mitigating symptoms and allowing patients to achieve their end-of-life goals. Preoperative planning for contingencies is a critical component of quality surgical care for patients with serious illness or high-stakes surgical problems. Regardless of the decision for or against operative intervention, efforts to maximize patient comfort, maintain dignity, and support efforts toward transcendence are core components of excellent surgical care and should be the focus of surgical teams working to help patients and their families achieve a positive end-of-life experience.

Takeaway Points

1. Surgery and palliative care can and should be integrated and concurrent, as opposed to mutually exclusive and sequential.
2. A key aspect of high-quality preoperative communication and decision-making is to focus on goals and values, rather than treatment preferences.
3. Required reconsideration is the preferred approach to handling advance directives including code status limitations perioperatively.
4. Control of nausea and vomiting due to benign and obstruction often requires multimodal approaches, including operative intervention if appropriate; a broad array of pharmacologic agents, including those that blunt central and peripheral nausea receptors and reduce gastrointestinal secretions; and enteral decompression. "Sometimes, the best palliative care is an operation." – *Anne Mosenthal, MD, FACS, October 2018.*

References

1. Cooper Z, Koritsanszky LA, Cauley CE, Frydman JL, Bernacki RE, Mosenthal AC, Gawande AA, Block SD. Recommendations for best communication practices to facilitate goal-concordant care for seriously ill older patients with emergency surgical conditions. Ann Surg. 2016;263(1):1–6.
2. Taylor LJ, Nabozny MJ, Steffens NM, Tucholka JL, Brasel KJ, Johnson SK, Zelenski A, Rathouz PJ, Zhao Q, Kwekkeboom KL, Campbell TC, Schwarze ML. A framework to improve surgeon communication in high-stakes surgical decisions: best case/worst case. JAMA Surg. 2017;152(6):531–8.
3. Urman RD, Lilley EJ, Changala M, Lindvall C, Hepner DL, Bader AM. A pilot study to evaluate compliance with guidelines for preprocedural reconsideration of code status limitations. J Palliat Med. 2018;21(8):1152–6.

Chapter 26
Geriatric Trauma Decision-Making Based on Functional Outcomes

David Zonies and Andrea K. Nagengast

Case Introduction

A 91-year-old female presents to the emergency department (ED) with intermediate-level trauma activation after being found down for an unknown length of time at the skilled nursing facility in which she resides. Although not witnessed, her mechanism of injury is presumed to be a ground-level fall. In the emergency room, she complains of head and back pain. She is mildly confused and scores 14 (Eye 4, Verbal 4, and Motor 6) on the Glasgow coma scale (GCS). Her physical exam is otherwise significant for left forehead swelling and ecchymosis.

Her trauma workup is completed and is notable for an acute subarachnoid hemorrhage and left maxillary sinus fracture on CT imaging of her head. She has a past medical history significant for paroxysmal supraventricular tachycardia and hypertension. In the ED, consults for trauma, neurosurgery, and facial trauma are placed.

Usual Approach

Falls are the leading cause of injury in geriatric trauma patients. One out of every three adults >65 will fall each year. By 2030, one in five Americans will be over age 65, and the population over age 85 is expected to double to nearly 12 million people by 2035. Frailty increases their risk and is the leading cause of traumatic brain injury in this group.

The patient is admitted to the ICU for hemodynamic and neurological monitoring. Delirium develops on hospital day 3 and the patient does not pass a swallow

D. Zonies (✉) · A. K. Nagengast
Department of Surgery, Oregon Health and Science University, Portland, OR, USA
e-mail: zonies@ohsu.edu

© Springer Nature Switzerland AG 2020
K. Aberger, D. Wang (eds.), *Palliative Skills for Frontline Clinicians*,
https://doi.org/10.1007/978-3-030-44414-3_26

evaluation. She has a waxing and waning mental status and a feeding tube is recommended for nutritional support. The patient is transferred to a skilled nursing facility. She is re-admitted to the ICU 3 days later for aspiration pneumonia and is intubated. The patient does not wean from the ventilator and the family withdraws life support. The patient dies in the ICU.

Palliative Approach

In the ED, you sit with the patient's daughter to find out more about the patient. The patient has been independent but in the last few months has slowed down. She is now confused at baseline. Her daughter informs you that her mother has a POLST (Physician Order For Life Sustaining Therapy). You review the document, which states DNR/DNI with limited additional interventions.

> **Box 26.1 POLST and Advance Directives**
> Early inquiry about a patient's POLST, Advance Directive, and code status is essential. If a patient is unable to provide the information and no family or surrogate is immediately available, perform a query of the state POLST registry if available. If your electronic health record is linked regionally, investigate to see if documents have been uploaded to neighboring hospitals.

The on-call neurosurgeon evaluates the patient, reviews her imaging studies, and recommends admission to the ICU for hourly neurologic checks. A repeat head CT with associated CTA is ordered for 6 hours after the initial imaging study. A coagulation panel is ordered and no correctable coagulopathy is noted. Twice daily dosing of Levatiracetam is scheduled for a total of 7 days, administered intravenously with planned transition to oral dosing after the patient is allowed a diet.

The on-call facial trauma resident evaluates the patient and reviews her imaging studies. Her case is staffed with the on-call attending and her maxillary sinus fracture is deemed non-operative. The facial trauma service signs off the patient's care and recommends follow-up in their outpatient clinic 2 weeks after discharge.

The patient's age (>80) will trigger an inpatient consult to the geriatric medicine team, who will assist with managing delirium, pain control, and continued discussions about goals of care.

Box 26.2 Geriatric Trauma Patients: A Palliative Centered Algorithm (Oregon Health and Science University, 2019)

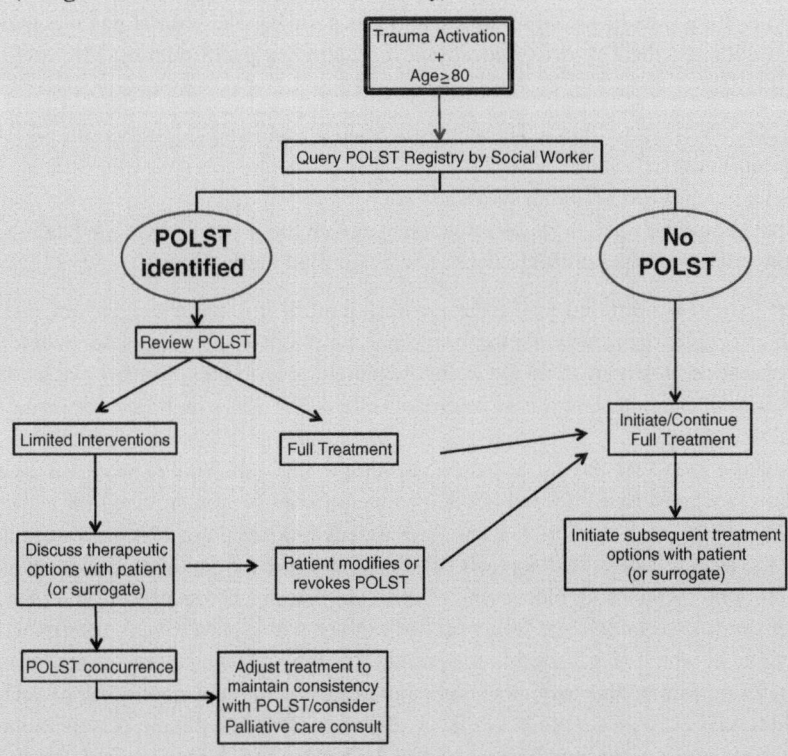

This framework not only navigates situations that fall outside of the norm for consulting services, but also encourages early, goal-directed discussions focused on ensuring the patient's wishes are honored.

It is important to discuss the extent of traumatic injuries with the patient or surrogate and share consulting services' plans or treatment. Rather than focusing the entirety of initial conversations on treatment options alone, talk with the patient or surrogate and work to identify what functional outcomes are acceptable. This conversation should happen as early as possible, while the patient is still in the emergency room, and helps guide overall care trajectory by allowing for early shared decision-making.

Communication with consulting services is essential, as this type of approach initially may be uncomfortable for some services. With thoughtful communication and thorough documentation, it is possible to treat the patient in line with individual goals of care.

Despite the consulting neurosurgical recommendations for admission to the ICU, you halt this planned disposition based on the conversations you have had with the patient's daughter in the ED. She reiterates that her mother would not want any invasive procedures; she has lived a full life and accepts when her natural death comes.

You consider the following questions in determining a thoughtful disposition from the ED:

- If not admitted to the ICU, what treatments and medical interventions are appropriate?
- Will a repeat head CT be necessary?
- What should be done if the bleed worsens, given the patient's POLST/AD?
- How often should neurologic checks be performed on the floor?

The patient is admitted to the floor with a goal of discharge as early as safely possible. You defer further imaging or regular neuro checks, since neither will lead to an operative intervention. In the event the patient deteriorates, you approach code status with her daughter by first referencing her POLST, which she confirms as DNR/DNI.

Over the next few days, the patient develops delirium. You manage this with small doses of psychotropics but her delirium continues to worsen. She fails a swallow study. After deliberation, her daughter agrees to a temporary NG feeding tube while the patient works with speech therapy. Days later, the patient fails a second swallow study and PEG placement is discussed with her daughter. Now given greater clinical certainty, she tells you her mother would never want a permanent feeding tube, which is reflected in the patient's POLST. You have a lengthy discussion with her about the patient's likely functional status and quality of life. Her daughter wishes for her mother's POLST to be honored. The patient is transitioned to comfort care and her daughter wants to take her home. The patient is discharged to her daughter's home with hospice services.

Box 26.3 Falls, Frailty, and Functional Outcomes

Falls are the leading cause of injury in geriatric trauma patients. One out of every three adults over age 65 will fall each year. Frailty is the leading cause of traumatic brain injury in falls. Mortality is not the only outcome that matters to these patients. Surveys have demonstrated that quality of life and independence are sometimes reported as even more important than prolonging life. Poor functional outcomes may be unacceptable for certain individuals and would, therefore, prompt a transition away from invasive procedures and toward comfort measures or hospice.

Take-Away Points

1. It is appropriate to slow down the admission process to allow time to establish goals of care based on patient preference, resuscitation status, and consistency with prior advanced directives and POLST forms in the geriatric trauma patient.
2. Use a framework which centers initial discussions with patients, caregivers, and designated surrogates about expected functional outcomes to assist in determining overall treatment plans, rather than basing initial discussions on treatment options alone.
3. Search the electronic medical record for advance care planning documents. Moreover, it is essential to thoroughly document any code status or goals of care discussion.
4. If a patient has a pre-existing POLST or a designated surrogate is identified AFTER hospital admission and this impacts the patient's level of care, ensure smooth transition to a level of care and treatment consistent with the patient's goals and values.

Part IV
Specialty Medicine

Chapter 27
Decision by Surrogates for a Patient with a Psychiatric History

Jennifer Y. Fung

Case Introduction

A 64-year-old woman with schizoaffective disorder and chronic obstructive pulmonary disease (COPD) is admitted with a COPD exacerbation. She has recently been a patient in the emergency department (ED) of a nearby hospital where she was told she had pneumonia, but she left against medical advice. In your ED, she informs the staff that she has been intubated before, and is supposed to be on oxygen at home. Shortly thereafter, she develops atrial fibrillation with rapid ventricular rate and respiratory distress, leading to intubation. Due to worsening hypotension, she is cardioverted twice, and central lines are placed emergently with initiation of vasopressors and continuous veno-venous hemofiltration (CVVH) due to acute kidney injury. Since no family has been located, she is presumed full code. Two physicians provide consent for the procedures.

Usual Approach

The patient receives full ICU support: antibiotics, pressors, and artificial ventilation. Because of her COPD history, she does not wean off of the ventilator. She progresses to tracheostomy, percutaneous gastrostomy tube, and LTACH placement. No next of kin are located, and the guardianship process is initiated.

J. Y. Fung (✉)
Department of Medicine, Mount Sinai Morningside, New York, NY, USA

© Springer Nature Switzerland AG 2020   189
K. Aberger, D. Wang (eds.), *Palliative Skills for Frontline Clinicians*,
https://doi.org/10.1007/978-3-030-44414-3_27

Palliative Approach

Although the patient is incapacitated, you make efforts to ascertain her functional baseline and support network. You discover that she lives in a supportive housing residence. You call and speak with the building manager who reports that the patient smoked heavily, mainly kept to herself, and is estranged from her family. He recalls that ambulances often came to pick the woman up, but that she would return days later saying she had walked out, saying "I know my body best."

> **Box 27.1 Preferences vs Capacity**
> In patients who lack capacity, whether from acute medical illness, mental illness, or other disability, the medical team should attempt to determine what the patient's values are and what would be important to them in terms of quality of life. Patients who have little capacity to make complex decisions may still express valuable preferences: "I don't want to be poked by needles," or "I would rather be home than in medical facilities." When patients cannot speak for themselves, it is important to obtain evidence of their preferences or wishes from others.

With the help of the housing contact, the ICU social worker is able to find her family. Over the next week, her sister and many cousins arrive from out of town. In this time, the patient improves moderately and is extubated. She informs the staff that she would agree to be intubated again, but does not want a tracheostomy or be on a ventilator indefinitely. Later in the night, she develops hypercapnic cardiac arrest, and recovers spontaneous circulation after 6 minutes. Following that resuscitation, she remains encephalopathic, with anuric renal failure, and becomes ventilator- and pressor-dependent.

You meet with the patient's sister and cousins. Before giving any medical information, you begin by asking them about the patient and what her life was like prior to this hospitalization.

Owing to her psychiatric history, the family had lost touch with her for many years. They were aware that she spent most of her time watching television and smoking cigarettes. One cousin knew that she had left the hospital against medical advice on multiple occasions in the past, inferring that she did not like being in a medical setting. They expressed their love for her but personal and emotional challenges made it difficult to interact with her.

With their permission, you provide a medical update, and note that the patient does not want to be on long-term mechanical ventilation. They are not surprised to hear this, and say, "That sounds just like something she would say." You minimize jargon and explain that she is "on full life support because all of her organs are in failure." While you could discuss each organ system in detail, it would detract their attention from the more important questions. You do acknowledge that tracheostomy may not be necessarily permanent for her.

Her family is appreciative, and they all defer to the patient's sister. While she knows that her sister's body has suffered many setbacks over the years, she "hopes that she will get better." You astutely ask, "What would getting better look like to her?"

Box 27.2 Getting Better – A Knee-Jerk Reflex
The complexity of ICU patients makes it difficult for families, even those with high health literacy, to understand the global picture. When multiple consultants are involved, often a given message that one organ system has improved will be extrapolated to include the entire clinical direction. Even "stable" carries a positive connotation. When prompted with the hope or belief that the patient is getting better, it is valuable to immediately follow up and ask them to elaborate on their impression of what is happening now, and their goal for what that may lead to.

Her sister hopes her sibling is able to return to her prior functional state, living in a long-term facility, and receiving occasional dialysis, if needed. You share your concerns that while the patient may be weaned off some of her current support, you do not believe she would return to her prior semi-independent state. Her family asks for time to deliberate amongst themselves.

The next day, the family members have decided they would like to proceed with tracheostomy. Her sister wishes to give the patient a chance to recover to her prior functional state. Although they know that most likely the patient will be limited, they do not believe this would necessarily be unacceptable to her. Her sister believes that living in a long-term care facility would not be that much different from the patient's current sedentary lifestyle and it would be consistent with her values. She also admits, and accepts, that some of this decision is as much for herself as it is for the patient. She feels guilt having been absent in her life, and now that they have reconnected, she intends to seize this opportunity to make amends.

Box 27.3 Prognosis Is About More than Communicating Knowledge
While clinicians place significant emphasis on accurately prognosticating and clearly communicating information, most surrogate decision-makers weigh their own experiences and values as heavily as they do your clinical expertise. Even when the transfer of prognostic knowledge is perfect, one-third of surrogates will be more optimistic than clinicians, commonly endorsing: a need to be hopeful for the patient or others, and a feeling that the patient is superior and unlike other patients in the same situation, with similar religious beliefs [1].

Hearing this juxtaposition between the sister's decision and the patient's own words, your team feels uncomfortable about this situation. Do you honor the patient's spoken wishes or the sister's hope? The physicians, nurses, respiratory therapists, and other staff collectively feel moral distress. You request an ethics committee consultation to evaluate what would be the most appropriate path forward.

The ethics committee weighs both the patient's autonomy as well as non-maleficence (non-harm). They are concerned that the patient may not have made a fully informed decision. Although her pattern of prior actions and behaviors suggests a disinterest in prolonged medicalization, she does seem to be enjoying her quality of life, and her agreement to reintubation supports this as well. Furthermore, in that moment, there is not enough demonstration over time to suggest if her schizoaffective disorder or residual toxic/metabolic encephalopathy has swayed her statements. Although autonomy is often given the greatest weight, in this instance, her ability to serve as her own agent is deemed less valuable than the maintenance of her life. Therefore, they conclude that it would be ethically appropriate to perform the tracheostomy, with the hope of returning the patient to a status where she could further voice her own wishes.

With this clarified, the patient's course is clear. The code status is reverted to full code. Hemodialysis is initiated. Tracheostomy and feeding tubes are placed. The patient's respiratory status improves and she can tolerate a trach collar for short periods of time. She is started on a puree diet while reducing tube feeds. She is able to mouth answers to simple questions, denying any discomfort or depression. However, she does not regain the capacity to make meaningfully complex decisions. She is discharged to a rehabilitation ventilator facility after a 7-week stay in the ICU.

Take-Away Points
1. Patients who lack complete medical decision-making capacity may nonetheless be able to provide valuable preferences. When no participation is possible, seek collateral evidence.
2. When surrogates state they hope or believe that the patient is getting better, reflexively ask them what "better" will look like.
3. Optimistic bias in prognostication is strongly rooted in surrogates' personal beliefs and values, irrespective of how well physicians may communicate their expertise.
4. Ethics consultation may be helpful when there is moral distress or discordance.

Reference

1. White DB, et al. Prevalence of and factors related to discordance about prognosis between physicians and surrogate decision makers of critically ill patients. JAMA. 2016;315(19):2086–94.

Chapter 28
Palliative Approach to Patients with Concurrent Serious Illness and Substance Use Disorder

Alison Petok and Brooke Worster

Case Introduction

A 28-year-old woman presents to the emergency department with increased pain and shortness of breath. She has stage III cervical cancer. However, she has not gone to see her physician for several months. Her cervical cancer has progressed on CT scan, with a large pelvic mass causing partial bladder and bowel obstruction. She also has pleural effusions. She is admitted for management of these complications. She is alternately tearful and angry when discussing potential treatments with the inpatient teams, including brachytherapy and XRT, and asks to be fully sedated to complete it. She insists on intravenous opioids for pain management, with increasing usage over the first 24 hours of her hospital stay. The nurses report that she seems sedated, but continues to ask for additional opioids, all the while complaining of extreme pain "all over."

Usual Approach

When patients exhibit drug-seeking behaviors, limits are often rapidly put in place, including strict avoidance of parenteral opioids and significant de-escalation of non-parenteral opioids. Often, this patient is discharged and readmitted within days or

A. Petok
Private Practice, Jamaica Plain, MA, USA

B. Worster (✉)
Department of Medical Oncology, Thomas Jefferson University Hospital/Sidney Kimmel Cancer Center, Philadelphia, PA, USA
e-mail: Brooke.Worster@jefferson.edu

© Springer Nature Switzerland AG 2020
K. Aberger, D. Wang (eds.), *Palliative Skills for Frontline Clinicians*,
https://doi.org/10.1007/978-3-030-44414-3_28

weeks due to uncontrolled pain or overdose. This burdensome, non-beneficial cycle typically continues for prolonged periods of time. The patient is labeled as "non-compliant" and "drug-seeking."

Palliative Approach

You find out more about the patient's social situation. The patient is here with her wife and her mother. She is also the primary caregiver for her wife who has multiple sclerosis. The patient has a complex social history, including ongoing poly-substance use disorder and years' long sexual trauma from childhood.

When meeting cancer patients, we often focus on the diagnosis and treatment of the disease. This focus and sense of urgency is often heightened when working with a patient such as this one, simultaneously facing cancer and serious SUD [1]. Asking about earlier abuse is rare in this setting, but it is not uncommon that many of our patients have a sexual trauma history and become re-traumatized by cancer treatments. In fact, many of the sterile clinical procedures gynecological cancer patients face tend to be similar in nature to their earlier trauma. For example, the treatment of this patient with radiation, brachytherapy, anesthesia, and surgery may include elements such as darkness, being silenced and immobilized, exposure of sexual organs, penetration, infliction of pain, and, ultimately, feeling as if she is under someone else's control and completely vulnerable [2].

Having a knowledgeable team, including social work, psychology, and palliative care, and taking a trauma-informed approach to care, can greatly improve the provider–patient relationship. Adults who were traumatized as children, as this patient was, can become stuck in fight or flight mode, or in chronic shutdown, and the right approaches are invaluable to providing their medical care [3]. In this case, we see the patient attempting to shut out *her* providers. She has most likely been coping with her trauma history over a number of years through drug use. Using a trauma-informed approach – acknowledging the potential for secondary traumatization and compassion fatigue, and providing self-care – can help build a relationship and also benefit providers.

The first step in providing a trauma-informed approach is to understand how to ask about past history of abuse [2]. (See the table below for more guidance on how to take a trauma history when meeting a patient.) Another key principle is collaboration and mutuality, or the idea that partnering can level the power differences between the health care team and the patient. Healing can occur in the context of a meaningful sharing of power and decision-making (Table 28.1).

Case Continued

A family meeting is held with the patient, her wife, and providers from oncology, social work, and palliative care, to discuss options for cancer care and acknowledge that she has real pain as well as ongoing SUD. There is a reasonable option of

Table 28.1 Exploratory questions in a trauma-informed approach

"I ask all my patients about prior or childhood trauma because unfortunately it does happen and it can impact your health."	Use attentive body language and be comfortable with silence.
"Has anyone ever done something sexual to you that you didn't want? Has anyone ever hit you or hurt you physically?"	Do not ask these questions in front of family or friends as it may make the patient uncomfortable to answer or potentially put them in an unsafe situation.
"I am asking you this because some people with a history of abuse may struggle with certain medical treatments. If we are aware of your history we can do a better job making this experience as comfortable as possible."	
"It sounds like that was really painful and scary. We are here to support you through this process and keep you safe."	Reflect back the emotions shared by the patient and convey support and respect for the patient.

continued opioid use, but it must be done in a manner that is not harmful. During the family meeting, the team learns that the patient has been selling some of her medications to obtain heroin, which she has been snorting. In that case, medication options of methadone or suboxone may be preferred over short-acting opiates alone. Social work support must be present to help connect with community-based SUD treatments. The patient also admits that in addition to the sexual abuse she experienced as a child, she also lived in unstable housing. Her father died of a drug overdose when she was very young; her mother exchanged sex for drugs. The patient first used heroin with her mother when she was 14 years old. She expresses fear of abandonment and mistrust of many individuals, including several team members involved in her care. A careful trauma-informed approach is used throughout the meeting.

During hospitalization, a multidisciplinary team decides that an opioid regimen of methadone 15 mg TID with non-opioid adjuvant medications, including NSAID and tricyclic antidepressant medications, are both efficacious and do the least harm. A psychiatrist who also specializes in SUD and operates the connected methadone maintenance program sees her during the hospitalization. He invites her to the program "as often as she can medically tolerate" and recommends behavioral monitoring with daily group therapy. He will also maintain communication with the palliative medicine physician who will directly manage all opioids. Finally, interventional radiology is consulted and performs a superior hypogastric plexus block to aid in pain relief before discharge.

Box 28.1 Importance of Shared Decision-Making (SDM) in Trauma-Informed Approach

Because the patient–physician relationship has traditionally been characterized by imbalances in power and knowledge, shared-decision making is another critical component of a trauma-informed approach. The discussion of SDM and patient-centered care appears ubiquitous in medicine, but is not practiced as routinely. This is partly due to apprehension on the part of patients to fully participate in their care in this way. It may also be due to misplaced expectations from clinicians. In substance use disorder, the concept of SDM deviates significantly from the more common concept of compliance [4]. In compliance, a provider determines a course of care to which they demand a patient adhere. In SDM, the provider and the patient must become joint experts in determining the optimal course of care. This means discussing treatment options as well as taking into account a full patient history, which includes their values and wishes. Although what is agreed upon may deviate from the optimal treatment course, providing choice and self-empowerment can both be incredibly powerful tools to individuals with mental illness or substance use disorder. Engaging a patient in decision-making in this context can also increase a sense of mastery or self-efficacy for the patient [5].

Forming a relationship built on mutual trust and understanding is critical to practicing true SDM. Another component on the side of the provider is understanding one's own values and recognizing them in oneself, but always allowing the patient's values to guide decision-making. SDM means working together to reach a mutually agreed upon decision.

Case Continued

After 3 months, the patient presents again to your ED with worsening pain and vaginal bleeding. She completed brachytherapy during her last admission, but ignored several subsequent appointments. She called the oncology office several times complaining of pain and demanding increased opioids, but did not follow instructions to come to the office or visit her local ED. At this point, the disease has spread extensively. She appears disheveled and cachectic. Upon conversation with gynecologic oncology, medical oncology, and palliative care, the risk of cytotoxic chemotherapy is felt to be greater than the benefit given her ECOG is 3. Her mother is no longer involved in her care.

She now complains of "all over pain" and requests higher doses of opioids. During the conversation, the wife asks to speak with the social worker privately. In this meeting, her wife reveals that the patient has continued to use heroin at home. She states that she is deeply saddened by the patient's continued drug use and has asked her to quit; she has done a great deal to provide support. The patient has also rejected several visits from the home nursing team. The patient, who knows her family does not want her to use drugs, has snuck out of the house late at night to acquire heroin. There is concern that she may be diverting her opioids in order to acquire drugs. The patient is unable to give a clear history of her medication usage. It is unclear if she understands the severity of her diagnosis.

Usual Approach

You consult GYN oncology and push for possible pelvic exenteration, restrict or completely limit opioids, and offer treatment for heroin use via methadone or suboxone therapy, and inpatient rehab or intensive outpatient rehab. She continues to appear detached during daily evaluations, and many nursing staff find caring for her personally distressing, their inherent compassion tempered by her "difficult" demeanor.

Palliative Approach

A repeat family meeting with goals of care conversation is held, including both the patient's support network and also hospital social work and chaplaincy. The patient admits that she has lost several family members in a traumatic fashion, including her cousin who was killed in a serious car accident, and she thinks of this often. Though she has acted nonchalant about death and dying in the past, she now opens up, offering glimpses of existential crises, including remorse for decisions she has made in the past. Although she wants to live, she understands that her cancer has become incurable. Considering the briefness of her life to date, this causes her significant emotional pain. Throughout the conversation, social work and chaplaincy help acknowledge, validate, and process her feelings.

You now understand better her goals *and* her needs. You recommend home hospice to provide optimal multidisciplinary support to her and her family as they continue their journey. The patient and her wife agree. She admits she is scared of withdrawal and dying in pain. You openly acknowledge without judgment the role that heroin abuse is playing in her plan of care. You also discuss how hospice can safely dispense opioids in a weekly fashion upon transition home. She is willing to do whatever is necessary to control both of these factors.

> **Box 28.2 Framework for Trauma-informed Goals of Care Meeting with Shared Decision-Making**
>
> Elicit the patient and family understanding of the current medical status.
>
> Acknowledge the patient's physical and emotional pain.
>
> Ask the patient more questions about her values related to EOL care; ask about fears and hopes and validate all feelings.
>
> Present all treatment options at this point in the trajectory of care using well-defined language and clearly discussing all benefits to each option.
>
> Empower the patient to make choices; be comfortable sitting with silence.
>
> Include social work and other members of the multidisciplinary team in GOC discussion.

Given her desire to cease heroin use and also avoid withdrawal, you recommend that the admitting team initiate medication-assisted treatment (MAT) using opioid substitution therapy, usually methadone or buprenorphine. MAT has been widely shown to be twice as effective as robust cessation programs without medication components. The admitting team inquires how a partial opioid agonist would impact their usual analgesic approach.

Box 28.3 Pain Management in the Setting of Opioid Use Disorder (OUD)

Initiation of medication-assisted treatment (MAT) with methadone or buprenorphine is preferred to prevent withdrawal or cravings. This is especially helpful as a patient functionally declines and may become physically unable to obtain heroin or illicit opioids. MAT medications bind with high affinity at the mu receptor, displacing effects from other prescription or illicit opioids, while also manifesting a partial agonist effect, thereby limiting euphoria and abuse.

Treatment of acute pain can be accomplished while receiving opioid agonist therapy. Due to tolerance and other factors, patients receiving maintenance therapy with opioids for addiction treatment do not derive sustained analgesia from it [6]. Buprenorphine is generally safely tolerated and has a ceiling effect on respiratory depression (does not proportionally increase with dosage). Risks for respiratory depression are usually not augmented by MAT medications themselves. Thus, the concern about severe drug toxicity with analgesic opioid treatment is not supported by clinical or empirical experience in patients on MAT with acute pain [7].

Use non-opioid adjuvants when possible and monitor for pain relief with these agents.

Utilize non-drug adjuvants whenever possible (i.e., relaxation techniques, acupuncture).

Work within interdisciplinary teams to ensure all aspects of pain addressed (social, emotional, spiritual).

Utilize pill counts and have a safe method to secure medications (lock box, family control).

If necessary, limit the amount of medication given at any one time (i.e., 1 week supply).

The patient is admitted for symptom control and hospice. She benefits from continued social work and chaplaincy visits. She is started on MAT with daily methadone for her OUD. With clear treatment goals for pain, her pain improves on daily incremental assessments and she arrives at a stable oral opioid regimen after a brief period on patient-controlled analgesia. She is also started on an anxiolytic, resulting in overall decreased opioid need. Days later, she is discharged home with hospice and is optimally managed at home without any further ED visits or hospitalizations.

Take-Away Points
1. Consider a trauma-informed approach, including patient-first shared decision-making, for serious illness patients with concurrent substance use disorder or who may be demonstrating behavioral challenges with their care plans.
2. A multidisciplinary team, including social work and chaplaincy, is essential in the process of listening to, collaborating with, and empowering patients in choices for their care.
3. Medication-assisted treatment with buprenorphine or methadone is a vital strategy in patients with substance use disorder, and should not interfere with their acute pain management.
4. Communicate care plans with hospice or outpatient programs so that they may continue to expertly manage symptoms while also safely dispensing opioids in these complex patients.

References

1. Lawson KC, Lawson DH. Insights into the psychology of trauma should inform the practice of oncology. Oncologist. 2018;23(7):750–1. https://doi.org/10.1634/theoncologist.2019-0091.
2. Schnur JB, Goldsmith RE. Through her eyes. J Clin Oncol. 2011;29(30):4054–6. https://doi.org/10.1200/JCO.2011.37.2409.
3. Van der Kolk B. The body keeps the score: brain, mind, and body in the healing of trauma. New York: Penguin Books; 2014.
4. Drake RE, Cimpean D, Torrey WC. Shared decision making in mental health: prospects for personalized medicine. Dialogues Clin Neurosci. 2009;11(4):455–63. Retrieved from https://www.ncbi.nlm.nih.gov/pmc/articles/PMC3181931/pdf/DialoguesClinNeurosci-11-455
5. Kon A. The shared decision-making continuum. JAMA. 2010;304(8):903–4.
6. Alford DP, Compton P, Samet JH. Acute pain management for patients receiving maintenance methadone or buprenorphine therapy. Ann Intern Med. 2006;144(2):127.
7. Lipman AG. Pain management, palliative care, and substance abuse. J Pain Palliat Care Pharmacother. 2012;26(2):96–7.

Chapter 29
Responding to Spiritual Suffering and Hope During a Goals-of-Care Conversation

Evan Wong

Introduction

This chapter presents communication skills to support medical providers of any discipline to respond to patients and families expressing religious and spiritual views in relation to their medical condition. It offers both an inner framework for managing one's own reactivity and an outer skillset for navigating the conversation. These tools enhance patient care in multiple ways: they build relationships; create the conditions for values-based, medically informed decision-making; support ongoing, mutual development of goals of care; and encourage meaning-making and well-being amidst the inevitable uncertainty, grief, and loss that are so common in palliative care.

The following three cases are from in-patient specialty palliative care, and take place between a patient/family and a palliative care chaplain. Each case will invoke principles that are valuable to any healthcare provider who cares for seriously ill patients and their families.

Case 1: When There Is Hope for a Miracle

Mr. D is a 68-year-old Chinese-American man. His wife is his primary decision-maker for healthcare, and they have two children in their 20s. Mr. D recently learned that he has metastatic cancer and that several organ systems are now failing. You approach the patient to discuss goals of care. Upon entering the room, the patient is asleep and his wife is at bedside. The patient identifies as Buddhist and his primary

E. Wong (✉)
Department of Palliative Care, Kaiser Permanente, Fremont, CA, USA
e-mail: evan.wong@berkeley.edu

© Springer Nature Switzerland AG 2020
K. Aberger, D. Wang (eds.), *Palliative Skills for Frontline Clinicians*,
https://doi.org/10.1007/978-3-030-44414-3_29

201

language is Cantonese. After introductions and a brief check-in, she begins by volunteering the following statement:

Mrs. D [With emotion] "He doesn't want to die. He's hoping for a miracle, you know."

You pause and first assess your own feelings. Recently you have been caring for many patients near their end of life, many whose care did not proceed as you would have imagined, and those experiences sit vividly in your memory. Noticing you are concerned that Mr. D will want full treatment and aggressive care at the end of his life, you recognize that it is important to put aside your views in service of the patient's autonomy in decision-making (*Manage inner reactivity/Intention*). You also notice your surprise that a Buddhist is hoping for a miracle since you are more familiar with your Christian patients using this term. You put these views aside as well, reminding yourself that each individual has their own way of connecting their beliefs to their experience and that "different words mean different things to different people." Aware of a subtle sense of anxiety about not knowing how this conversation will unfold, you manage your inner reactivity by taking a deep breath and feeling your feet on the floor before focusing your attention on Mrs. D (*Presence*).

Box 29.1 Inner Foundations

This inner skillset is essential for communicating with people with different views, and/or when there is a strong emotional component:

Presence: Offer the patient/family your full attention.

Manage inner reactivity: Know your biases as well as possible, put your views aside, recognize your reactivity in the moment, and self-soothe as necessary.

Intention: Be clear about where you want to be coming from, e.g., a desire to support autonomy in decision-making, to hold space for the patient/family's emotional state, or another such clear and helpful intention.

After using inner foundations to ground yourself, you seek first to understand before giving information. You look at Mrs. D and nod to *affirm* her experience, [thinking] "Mrs. D is expressing something that matters a lot to Mr. D and this deserves attention." To *learn more*, you inquire:

You "I see. What kind of miracle is he hoping for?"

Mrs. D "Just for more time. His friends have told him about other people with cancer who were diagnosed years ago and are still doing fine today."

You [Offering another *reflection*] "Ah, so he's hoping for more time, maybe even more years."

Mrs. D "Yes, I know it's not likely, but his mindset is the most important thing. Who am I to take away his hope?"

> **Box 29.2 Outer Skillset: AMEN Communication Protocol for Miracles**
> In response to the hope for miracles, the AMEN protocol (Affirm, Meet, Educate, No matter what) is a powerful tool to keep the conversation going rather than attempt to "solve an issue" [1]. It supports goals-of-care conversations to evolve incrementally, rather than all at once. This protocol has been built upon here to offer more detail and tools for working with patient/family religious beliefs in general.
>
> *Affirm/Meet and Reflect*: Demonstrate respect and communicate empathy for what the patient/family values and wants.
>
> *Learn more*: Get curious and ask to hear more about the miracle, hopes, or values framed through patient/family religious beliefs.
>
> *Broaden the care plan*: Determine what else is important so you can discuss different care plan options from the perspective of patient/family values and goals.
>
> *Educate* about the medical situation and options.
>
> *No matter what*: reassure the family you will support them no matter what happens. This promotes trust and leaves room for patient/family goals to change within your relationship.
>
> By demonstrating empathy at the beginning, learning more about what is important to a patient/family, and then broadening the care plan, you can assess a patient/family's needs, hopes, and worries. Then, when you later discuss the medical situation and options, you can more easily frame them in terms of how they align with patient/family values.

You   "His mindset is important and we definitely want to support that (*Affirm/ Meet/Reflect*). In addition to hope, what else is important to him right now?" (*Broaden the care plan*).

Mrs. D   "Just to be comfortable, for us to be here, to have time to rest."

You   "That's important for us too (*Meet*). Is there anything else we can do to help him with those things?"

Mrs. D   "No, everything is ok."

You   "I'm glad to hear that. I'm also hoping for the best and that Mr. D has as much time with you as possible." (*Affirm/Meet/Reflect*) [You wait to see if or how she responds, then notice Mrs. D take a deeper breath that gives you the sense that your reflection provided some relief. You also want to make sure you talk about other scenarios.] "If he were to get sicker, it's really important for us to have a plan (*Broaden the care plan*). I'd like to come back a little later with my colleagues to talk with Mr. D when he's awake. When do you think would be a good time?"

Later in the day, you and the entire palliative team visit Mr. and Mrs. D, and their two children with a Cantonese Interpreter. You acknowledge Mr. D's hope for more time and join him in hoping for that too. You also discuss the possibility of Mr. D getting sicker. You then work together to come up with a plan that allows for the possibility of Mr. D to get a bit better (continuing selective treatment) while also considering what his time may look like if he gets worse. Exploring this further, you help the family define what quality time would look like, and collectively agree to promote Mr. D's value for comfort, rest, and time with family by avoiding ICU-level care and CPR. You thank Mr. D and family for their willingness to have the conversation and affirm that you will support Mr. D and family no matter what happens.

Box 29.3 Reflection

Respecting and affirming Mrs. D's wish to support the patient's hopes allows her to trust her clinical team, and apply her energy for advocacy toward creating common goals and supporting her family rather than potentially resisting the clinical team. Taking time to build trust creates the foundation for open communication that leads to robust informed decision-making about goals of care. In one study, the medical professionals interviewed were three times less likely to believe in miracles than the general public [2]. Since healthcare providers frequently encounter patients and family members with beliefs and values different from their own, the inner foundation for managing one's own reactivity is an important tool for goals of care conversations.

Box 29.4 How Do Miracles Play Into Your Practice?

Here are some questions to ask yourself or discuss with others in order to support awareness of one's inner landscape and develop more facility in engaging with the hope for a miracle:

What are my thoughts about miracles?

What do I consider to be a miracle? Do they occur?

What judgments or reactions (if any) arise when a patient or family member says something about miracles or their religious beliefs?

How do I feel when a family makes a choice that I do not agree with? Is there a way for me to soothe these feelings and come to a place of acceptance of the patient/family wishes?

When I get irritated, frustrated, or unsure of what to say, what does that tend to look like in my communication? What do I need to do to return to a state of presence and acceptance?

Case 2: When Strong Religious Language Enters the Conversation

Mrs. F is an 84-year-old African-American woman. She has COPD and heart disease and was admitted to the hospital for shortness of breath associated with pneumonia. Mrs. F has been hospitalized multiple times over the past 3 months for breathing problems, staying in skilled nursing facilities between admissions for rehabilitation. She is currently requiring BiPAP. Two of the patient's children at bedside are listed as her primary and secondary decision-makers on her Advance Healthcare Directive, which indicates that the patient would desire life-prolonging measures in all medical circumstances. The patient and family identify as members of the Church of Christ.

After introductions, one of the daughters states the following:

Daughter   "We believe God knows everything about us. He knows when we were born and he knows when we will die. He created all the doctors and the medicine, and He created all the machines."

You notice your uncertainty about how you are going to find your way through this goals-of-care discussion as you do not know how the daughter's statement will impact decision-making. To support *presence* and *manage inner reactivity*, you take a breath and feel the sensations of your physical self. Then, you recall your *intention*: you want to understand more about what is important for this family and see where it progresses. You decide to *affirm* what the daughter has shared.

You   "It sounds like you have a very strong faith. I'm curious, how does your faith guide you with medical decisions?" *(Learn more)*.

Box 29.5 What Spiritual Care Can Teach Us About Palliative Care Communication

Spiritual care is not limited to the religious elements of a goals-of-care conversation. You offer spiritual care any time you listen to a patient/family explore why something is important to them, build relationships based on trust, humility, and acceptance, and honor their hopes, worries, and loss with kindness and respect.

Daughter   "The most important thing for us is to follow her wishes. She had said she wants us to give her every chance to live and that's what we're doing."

You   "I really admire your dedication to her and your support for her wishes. *(Affirm/Meet/Reflect)* In addition to giving her every chance to live, what else is important to her?" *(Broaden the care plan)*.

Daughter   "She really wants to go home. It's also really hard for us to see her not being able to eat because of the breathing mask."

You   *(Reflecting)* "So going home is important, and being able to eat?"

Daughter   "Yes, of course."

You   [Inviting a transition to *educate* about medical situation and options,] "Sometimes people's medical choices change over time as their medical conditions change. I think it could be helpful for our team to talk with you a bit more about your mother's medical condition so that we can work together to decide how to move forward while honoring your mother's wishes. Would that be ok?"

Daughter   "Yes, can we talk tomorrow? Hopefully she'll feel a bit better and be able to tell us what to do."

The next day, Mrs. F is in impending respiratory failure and unable to discuss her medical wishes. Your team helps the patient's daughters weigh the importance of honoring their mother's wishes against the prospect of likely not being able to return home or eat on her own again. Her daughters appreciate your consideration of their feelings, understand the gravity of their mother's situation, and choose to proceed with intubation to give the patient any possible chance to recover. They tell your team that they will know when it is time to shift to a comfort approach. After 1 week of intubation, tracheostomy is raised. They remember your conversation, and knowing now that those broader goals will not be achieved, they transition her to comfort care with a clear conscience, knowing they stayed true to their mother throughout this process.

> **Box 29.6 Reflection**
> Honoring the family's religious views and asking how these views influence medical decision-making revealed that the most important thing for the family was to honor the patient's wishes, not necessarily recovery. Sometimes a successful outcome for a family is less about what happens medically, and more about the meaning behind their medical decisions (in this case, staying true to the relationship they have had with their mother).

Case 3: When There Is Spiritual Distress

Mr. N is a multiracial man in his mid-40s. He has end-stage renal disease and heart failure, and began hemodialysis a few months ago, at which time the nephrologist cautioned him with a prognosis of "less than a year." Since then, he has had multiple hospitalizations with complications including infections and failure to thrive. He is transferred to the ICU this morning with a new pressor requirement. Mr. N is full code and he wants to "keep fighting." Multiple providers have attempted to change his code status, and he has become increasingly frustrated.

Your nurse suggests to you that a conversation with chaplaincy may be helpful. Since the patient is being followed by palliative care, you refer to the palliative care chaplain rather than the acute care chaplain.

You speak with the palliative care chaplain beforehand, noting your concerns about his worsening illness, and wish to discuss goals of care without further alienating him. The palliative care chaplain appreciates your coordination.

The palliative care chaplain meets with the patient, who is tearful on her arrival. After introductions, she asks him what is on his mind.

Box 29.7 Existential Distress Impacts the Care Plan and Patient/Family Wellbeing

Patients may share, and be receptive to, certain conversations with chaplains that they would not be in response to a provider. Although many palliative care teams do not yet have a dedicated chaplain on their service, referring cases to chaplains to assess and address existential needs, obtaining the chaplain's perspectives, and sharing the medical team's concerns with chaplains, can result in better patient care and overcoming impasses.

Mr. N	"I just don't know why this is happening to me."
PC Chaplain	[Takes a breath to pause and settle into her seat, supporting *presence*,] "Sounds like you're searching for some answers." (*Affirm/ Meet/Reflect*).
Mr. N	"Yeah, I want some answers! I want to ask the man upstairs, whoever that is, but first I'm going to beat him up! [With some tears] I'm not ready to go. There are still so many things I want to do."
PC Chaplain	[*Reflecting* back using simple words to open up the conversation without over-assuming] "I hear your frustration about not knowing why this is happening, and also some sadness."

She sits quietly at Mr. N's bedside, feeling compassion for his sadness and anger. From this point forward, the visit moves into a deeper exploration of the patient's emotional and spiritual needs in relation to his prognosis. She normalizes the variety of Mr. N's feelings, encourages him to express his anger "to the man upstairs," and offers a prayer at his request. Eventually, Mr. N shares that the most important thing for him is his family, and to "keep fighting to be with them." She *affirms* Mr. N's values and assures him that his teams will continue to support him in his journey.

After debriefing this exchange, you and the palliative care chaplain decide to round on Mr. N together each morning. Over the coming days, Mr. N expresses that although he does not understand why this is happening to him, the very act of committing to fighting for his life in order to show his family how much he loves them provides him with an important sense of agency when much of his life is no longer in his control. He opens up more and more, regularly grieving the losses in his mobility and identity as a "provider for my family." During one visit, Mr. N shares that while he will continue to fight as long as he can, that if the time ever comes when he can no longer communicate with his family, then he would want to have a peaceful death. Eventually Mr. N becomes intubated. His family, who initially are divided on how long to keep pressing onward with care, deeply appreciate when you share his own words with them. They feel a great weight is lifted from their shoulders and they transition him to comfort care days later. They share that they feel confident that Mr. N died "as a fighter" and "dedicated to his family," and made his exit on his own terms.

Box 29.8 Reflection

Although chaplains specialize in the spiritual and existential aspects of care, it is helpful for all medical providers to have some training and facility in addressing general spiritual issues. Patients and families have reported that it is appropriate for physicians to speak with them about their spiritual needs, although this is seldom done [3]. In addition to providing generalist spiritual care, collaborate with, and refer to, professional chaplains whenever spiritual issues arise so they may help to deepen the team's understanding of the patient's goals of care, provide spiritual support, and promote wellbeing.

Examples of spiritual issues include the following: patient needs additional emotional support; patient is trying to make sense of what is happening; patient has cultural and/or religious concerns and needs.

Regardless of whether the patient/family changes their mind about their goals of care, how you communicate matters. For example, offering time for family members to ask questions, express concerns, and confront painful emotions with supportive listening and discussion can have positive impacts on their bereavement and long-term mental health [4, 5].

Takeaway Points for Responding Skillfully When the Patient/Family Is in Spiritual Distress or Has a Different World View

1. Lay the groundwork by exploring your biases ahead of time. Practice returning to a state of presence and acceptance when triggered.
2. When spiritual language or hope for a miracle arises, use these as cues to deepen your relationship with the patient/family.
3. Align with the patient/family by reflecting and affirming their values. Be inquisitive and learn more by asking open-ended questions.
4. Broaden the care plan, exploring specific options that align with the patient/family's values.

References

1. Jacobs LM, Burns K, Bennett JB. Trauma death: views of the public and trauma professionals on death and dying from injuries. Arch Surg. 2008;143:730–5.
2. Lautrette A, Darmon M, Megarbane B, et al. A communication strategy and brochure for relatives of patients dying in the ICU. N Engl J Med. 2007;356:469–78.
3. Astrow AB, Wexler A, Texeira K, Kai He MK, Sulmasy DP. Is failure to meet spiritual needs associated with cancer patients' perceptions of quality of care and satisfaction with care? J Clin Oncol. 2007;25(36):5753–7.
4. Cooper RS, Ferguson A, Bodurtha JN, Smith TJ. AMEN in challenging conversations: bridging the gaps between faith, hope, and medicine. J Oncol Pract. 2014; 10(4): e191–e195.
5. Curtis JB, White DB. Practical guidance for evidence-based ICU family conferences. Chest. 2008;134:835–843.

Chapter 30
Trisomy 18: Early and Concurrent Palliative Care Enhances Delivery and Neonatal Planning

Nathan M. Riley, Ann Marie Case, Josephine Amory, and Krishelle Marc-Aurele

Case Introduction

A 45-year-old G5P3 female presents for prenatal care with an unplanned pregnancy. She has three healthy living children ages seven, ten, and twelve. Her fourth pregnancy ended in a second trimester miscarriage. In this pregnancy, she declined non-invasive prenatal screening. A formal anatomic survey in the second trimester revealed a cleft lip and palate, bilateral clubfeet, large ventricular septal defect, large omphalocele, intracranial findings suggestive of a Dandy Walker malformation, single umbilical artery, and mild bilateral renal pyelectasis. Diagnostic testing by amniocentesis now confirms a male fetus with Trisomy 18 (T18).

The patient and her partner are devout Catholics and consider every pregnancy a blessing. The loss of their fourth pregnancy at 20 weeks of gestation was devastating for them. They have some experience with special needs' parenting, as their friend gave birth prematurely at 25 weeks, and the newborn had an extensive stay in the neonatal intensive care unit (NICU). That child, now 8 years old, has cerebral palsy and requires assistance with all daily tasks.

N. M. Riley (✉)
Obstetrics and Gynecology, Palliative Medicine, Norton Healthcare, Louisville, KY, USA

A. M. Case
Pediatrics, Palliative Medicine, Dell Children's Medical Center of Central Texas, Austin, TX, USA

J. Amory
Maternal Fetal Medicine, Palliative Medicine, University of Washington, Seattle, WA, USA

K. Marc-Aurele
Neonatology, Palliative Medicine, University of California, San Diego, CA, USA

© Springer Nature Switzerland AG 2020   209
K. Aberger, D. Wang (eds.), *Palliative Skills for Frontline Clinicians*,
https://doi.org/10.1007/978-3-030-44414-3_30

Usual Approach

A T18 diagnosis generally prompts referral to a maternal fetal medicine specialist (MFM). The MFM performs a detailed ultrasound to confirm the findings, offers diagnostic testing such as amniocentesis, and may refer the patient to a genetics counselor for a thorough explanation of the diagnosis and review of recurrence risk for future pregnancies. In the case of T18, the MFM provides management options – expectant management or termination of pregnancy – with an explanation of relevant risks and benefits after confirming the diagnosis. This discussion includes the possibility of miscarriage or intrauterine fetal demise, as well as likelihood of the newborn's survival after birth. Referral to an MFM may take up to two weeks to get the visit authorized and scheduled. Full diagnostic work-up may necessitate several more weeks thereafter.

If the patient chooses to terminate the pregnancy, the MFM provides counseling on medical or procedural management. If the patient chooses expectant management, she may be followed by her prenatal care provider with occasional follow-up visits with the MFM. If cardiac, neurologic, or other significant fetal anomalies are found that might require surgical intervention early in the infant's life, prenatal consultations with pediatric subspecialists are often included in order to educate the family around the risks and benefits of specific surgical interventions.

Frequently, the parents' concerns and hopes for a T18 newborn with anticipated comorbidities are not fully addressed. Consultation with a neonatologist typically happens in the third trimester. This reduces the time for the family to develop a trusting relationship with the team who will ultimately care for their child. Furthermore, birth planning, which is not guided by a goals-of-care discussion from the time of diagnosis, will not begin until late in the third trimester.

Palliative Approach

The patient is referred to a multidisciplinary team ideally at the time of diagnosis of a life-limiting newborn illness [1–3]. The optimal team includes a social worker with palliative skills, a chaplain, and a specialist in child-life services in addition to the obstetrician, MFM, neonatology team, and any additional pediatric or surgical specialists who may be involved after delivery. Even if the family does not identify with a particular faith, a chaplain on the team is present to address possible spiritual needs. Referrals to neonatology and pediatric palliative care are ideally placed shortly after diagnosis. Pediatricians are well-equipped to elaborate on the short- and long-term outcomes for newborns with T18. Early integration of a pediatric palliative care team, in particular, allows for continuity in goals-of-care assessment and family-centered planning beyond the perinatal period [4, 5]. This discussion elaborates on the family's values, religious and spiritual beliefs, and cultural practices, which inform decision-making around the complex prenatal diagnosis. From here, the multidisciplinary team helps align the parents' decisions with their values and goals of care for the child [6–8]. Delays in referral to this multidisciplinary team may result in lost opportunities to help parents process the diagnosis, prognosis, and management options as well as to provide needed support [9].

Box 30.1 Palliative Considerations at the Time of a Complex Prenatal Diagnosis

– Clear communication of diagnosis and prognosis tailored to the parents' needs after assessing what parents already know and what they want to know
– Use of primary palliative communication skills and early referral by the prenatal care provider to MFM, neonatology, and specialty palliative care as available
– Sensitive and nondirective exploration of pregnancy management options after exploration of the family's hopes and concerns
– Multidisciplinary team approach to help with elicitation of the family's values and beliefs in order to explore ongoing goals of care
– Observance of the importance of memory-making and spiritual practices during pregnancy and after birth
– Use of terms such as "baby" or a name chosen by the parents to align with the family and honor the pregnancy

---

Obstetricians, midwives, and other prenatal care providers play a particularly important role in coordinating family-centered care for the newborn. Regardless of their decision to continue the pregnancy, these parents have experienced a life-altering diagnosis and would benefit from palliative support. With a palliative approach, parents' perspective on the potential outcomes for their baby and family inform the goals of care. Discussing these hopes, wishes, and concerns is thus fundamental in providing the best family-centered care possible. Furthermore, parents' perception of their child's end-of-life care can factor into the risk for decisional regret and complicated grief [10].

Due to both better clinical awareness and advances in life-prolonging therapies, such as long-term artificial nutrition and cardiac surgical intervention, T18 is no longer characterized a terminal diagnosis, though it is still considered life-limiting and life-altering [11, 12]. Many parents subsequent to this diagnosis opt for termination of pregnancy, in which case their prenatal care providers' support is essential. Hospital and clinic staff should be mindful not to allow their own values to influence their ability to provide compassionate care for parents making this difficult decision [13]. Additionally, the obstetric team needs training on how language impacts parents' coping and grief [14]. It is best to avoid phrases such as, "At least you have your other children", "He is in a better place", "You can always have another baby", or "If I were in your situation, I would…".

Unfortunately, a newborn with T18 is at significant risk of death in the first year of life and beyond [15–18], although recent data suggest a much higher likelihood of longer-term survival if the infant survives beyond 6–12 months of life [19, 20]. In the event that the infant survives to be discharged from the NICU, the parents can be counseled that he is likely to have significant limitations related to feeding, mobility, speech, and social interaction [21]. A nuanced understanding of the parents' greatest concerns and their range of hopes – rather than a laundry list of the interventions they want or do not want – will allow the newborn team to guide family-centered decisions.

Box 30.2 Eliciting a Family's Values and Beliefs in Order to Facilitate a Meaningful Goals-of-Care Discussion

– To normalize the discussion, consider speaking in the third person: "For some families, their faith is really important when they make medical decisions. Is that the case for you?"
– To generalize the discussion, consider using a different sex of the baby in the examples you use of what other families have chosen
– "Given that your baby's time may be limited after birth, what are some things that are important to you for your baby when he comes into this world?"
– "What is most important when you think about your baby's future?"
– "For some families, because of their faith or culture, life is the most important priority. For other families, there may be things that are worse than death, like disability. What does your family think about this?"
– "What are you hoping for after he is born? What other hopes do you have?"

It is important that providers understand the parents' perspective on "good parenting." Parents should feel that they have been given realistic choices as well as guidance based on their personal goals and not a predetermined plan of care. Giving them time to contemplate these decisions and permission to change them is important. In some circumstances, it can also be helpful to outline a scenario of the "default" care that can be expected in the event that no decision is made prior to birth. [9, 13].

Delivery and neonatal planning is a critical component of ongoing counseling. Many parents elect life-prolonging interventions or a time-limited trial of intervention [20]. Comfort-focused care after a live birth is a reasonable alternative to intervention [22]. While "comfort-focused care" is a familiar phrase for care providers, it can be confusing for parents, so discussing what it entails ahead of time helps avoid misunderstandings after birth. Parents may initially choose it to maximize family time and then find that they desire feeding support for their infant after birth. If comfort-focused care is elected, it is essential to determine where the parents want to spend the baby's final moments of life. If the newborn lives beyond his expected prognosis, realistic options can be discussed. It may be helpful to introduce local hospice services when transfer to home is needed. Possible survival beyond the perinatal period should also be explored, as well as options for standard pediatric care for infants with chronic conditions, including referrals to pediatric specialists, therapists, and home health nursing. Throughout this process, provider flexibility – shown by asking permission, checking for understanding, and read-dressing goals of care – is vital.

Box 30.3 Birth Planning Considerations

- Intermittent versus continuous versus no fetal monitoring during labor
- Pain management for the mother to allow for maximum relief but also to allow her to stay alert to enjoy her time with her baby
- Clear plan for neonatal team to either provide resuscitation or to allow a natural death
- Preparing the parents and family members for the active dying process when you are not certain about the outcome
- Clear plan for the baby to stay with parents or to be transferred to the NICU
- Clear plan to identify which team (e.g., obstetric, NICU, etc.) will be responsible for the baby
- Pain, anxiety, and anti-seizure symptom management plans for the baby
- Special visitation plans for extended family or young siblings on labor and delivery unit or in the NICU
- Early communication with the chaplain or family's spiritual advisor
- Memory-making, including early communication with a specialized birth photographer (nonprofits such as *Now I Lay Me Down to Sleep* can provide these services free of charge)
- Preparation of nursing and other staff for conceivable outcomes
- If the obstetric team is managing the infant, a clear plan for transition to the pediatric team for routine care and discharge planning if extended survival is expected
- Consultation with pediatric palliative care and hospice providers if applicable

---

Follow-up visits with neonatology and relevant pediatric specialists will help guide parents' decision-making as the pregnancy progresses [23]. Regardless of which pregnancy management decision parents make, obstetricians, midwives, and doulas can assist with creating remembrances through encouraging family photos during the patient's pregnancy, or recording fetal heartbeat during prenatal visits. Bear in mind that multiple conversations are often required over the course of the pregnancy. Parents' grief processes are individualized, and their goals of care may evolve as they process the diagnosis and prognosis over time [24]. In facilitating these ongoing conversations, it is important to remember, as eloquently stated by Kiman and Doumac, that ...*bereavement can be an ongoing, continual process throughout the disease course. In this paradigm, healing and bereavement are facilitated with a mindset of 'being with', while curing is facilitated with the usual mindset of 'doing to'* [8, 25].

Apart from logistical birth planning, many parents fear the dying process and thus may benefit from a description of it. If there is a high risk for neonatal death at the time of birth, the labor and delivery staff should be prepared for this possibility and briefed on phrases and actions that may be soothing or distressing to the parents [26]. Phrases such as "We want to help you in any way we can. What else can we do to help you deal with this difficult situation?" and "You are brave and loving parents" are helpful [27]. Many parents have reported in retrospect that finding normalcy was of high importance. Some examples of activities that may promote normalcy include dressing their baby in family heirloom clothing, holding the baby, bathing or combing the baby's hair, taking photos, or performing a ceremony or ritual. In the immediate neonatal period, social support groups can be highly effective in providing parents with coping strategies during prolonged NICU stays or in the event of neonatal death [28]. When faced with a fetal diagnosis of T18, prenatal care providers should implement a palliative approach with early involvement of pediatric palliative specialists to coordinate complex care teams, advance care planning, and psychosocial-spiritual support throughout the pregnancy, child's lifespan, and over changing locations of care.

Case Conclusion

This patient ultimately opted to proceed with the pregnancy to birth. She was seen by a pediatric palliative care physician shortly after the diagnosis was confirmed by the MFM. Initially, she was only interested in "positive language" as it pertained to the possible outcomes of her pregnancy; however, as the pregnancy progressed and additional features of her baby's anatomy were elaborated, she began inquiring about the comfort-focused option. Involvement of a pediatric cardiac surgeon was important throughout this process, as he provided a critical piece of counseling throughout the patient's prenatal course. Serial ultrasounds revealed a severe cardiac defect that would require extensive surgery. Because the surgeon declined to offer heart surgery, the family decided that they would prefer "to leave matters in God's hands" and designed a comfort-focused birth plan with the help of the patient's obstetrician. The patient and her husband arranged for a maternity photoshoot, and they began a scrapbook with numerous ultrasound photos. The husband found it particularly difficult to face the reality that his son may die shortly after birth. He often asked questions like, "Why would God let this happen to my boy?" Our team's social worker was able to connect him and his wife with a support group for other families that have had to cope with life-limiting diagnoses, and our chaplain met with them additionally to address their spiritual concerns and to help them make meaning of this journey.

Prior to the patient going into labor, the labor and delivery and pediatrics staff were briefed on appropriate phrases in order to comfort the family in their time of grief. Ultimately, the patient gave birth in a private labor and delivery suite that was remote from other laboring patients. As expected, the newborn had irregular breathing and displayed cyanosis soon after delivery. The newborn was handed directly to his mother, and the family took photos and sang to him. He appeared comfortable with a smooth brow and was soothed by holding and swaddling. The newborn died at four hours of life with progressive apnea. A photographer from Now I Lay Me Down to Sleep arrived shortly thereafter to document the family in their time of mourning. The photographer captured valued photos of their newborn that would later be added to the family's scrapbook. The family was permitted to stay with the infant overnight in a private room remote from other families and newborns. After discharge from the hospital, the family continued to meet with a support group, which became a source of support throughout the grieving process.

> **Take-Away Points**
> 1. Complex prenatal diagnoses require multiple specialists to meet family needs and is best delivered through a multidisciplinary model.
> 2. A palliative approach seeks to obtain an understanding of parents' values, beliefs, and spiritual and cultural perceptions, which are critical to facilitating medical decision-making conversations around complex prenatal diagnoses.
> 3. Memory-making and support for the family should begin early in pregnancy and continue throughout the immediate neonatal period into childhood.
> 4. Discussion points from this perinatology case are widely applicable across a variety of complex prenatal and pediatric scenarios.

References

1. Twamley K, Craig F, Kelly P, Hollowell DR, Mendoza P, Bluebond-Langner M. Underlying barriers to referral to paediatric palliative care services: knowledge and attitudes of health care professionals in a paediatric tertiary care centre in the United Kingdom. J Child Health Care. 2014;18(1):19–30.
2. Thompson LA, Knapp C, Madden V, Shenkman E. Pediatricians' perceptions of and preferred timing for pediatric palliative care. Pediatrics. 2009;123(5):e777–82.
3. Haug S, Goldstein M, Cummins D, Fayard E, Merritt TA. Using patient-centered care after a prenatal diagnosis of trisomy 18 or trisomy 13: a review. JAMA Pediatr. 2017;171(4):382–7.
4. Marc-Aurele KL, Hull AD, Jones MC, Pretorius DH. A fetal diagnostic center's referral rate for perinatal palliative care. Ann Palliat Med. 2018;7(2):177–85.
5. Hasegawa SL, Fry JT. Moving toward a shared process: the impact of parent experiences on perinatal palliative care. Semin Perinatol. 2017;41(2):95–100.
6. Balaguer A, Martín-Ancel A, Ortigoza-Escobar D, Escribano J, Argemi J. The model of palliative care in the perinatal setting: a review of the literature. BMC Pediatr. 2012;12:25.
7. Calhoun BD. Perinatal hospice: compassionate and comprehensive care for families with lethal prenatal diagnosis. Linacre Q. 2010;77(2):147–56.
8. Kiman R, Doumic L. Perinatal palliative care: a developing specialty. Int J Palliat Nurs. 2014;20(3):143–8.
9. Andrews SE, Downey AG, Showalter DS, Fitzgerald H, Showalter VP, Carey JC, et al. Shared decision making and the pathways approach in the prenatal and postnatal management of the trisomy 13 and trisomy 18 syndromes. Am J Med Genet C: Semin Med Genet. 2016;172(3):257–63.

10. Tan JS, Docherty SL, Barfield R, Brandon DH. Addressing parental bereavement support needs at the end of life for infants with complex chronic conditions. J Palliat Med. 2012;15(5):579–84.
11. Janvier A, Farlow B, Wilfond BS. The experience of families with children with trisomy 13 and 18 in social networks. Pediatrics. 2012;130(2):293–8.
12. Morris JK, Savva GM. The risk of fetal loss following a prenatal diagnosis of trisomy 13 or trisomy 18. Am J Med Genet A. 2008;146A(7):827–32.
13. Henley A, Schott J. The death of a baby before, during or shortly after birth: good practice from the parents' perspective. Semin Fetal Neonatal Med. 2008;13(5):325–8.
14. Walker LV, Miller VJ, Dalton VK. The health-care experiences of families given the prenatal diagnosis of trisomy 18. J Perinatol. 2008;28(1):12–9.
15. Rasmussen SA, Wong L-YC, Yang Q, May KM, Friedman JM. Population-based analyses of mortality in trisomy 13 and trisomy 18. Pediatrics. 2003;111(4 Pt 1):777–84.
16. Vendola C, Canfield M, Daiger SP, Gambello M, Hashmi SS, King T, et al. Survival of Texas infants born with trisomies 21, 18, and 13. Am J Med Genet A. 2010;152A(2):360–6.
17. Brewer CM, Holloway SH, Stone DH, Carothers AD, FitzPatrick DR. Survival in trisomy 13 and trisomy 18 cases ascertained from population based registers. J Med Genet. 2002;39(9):e54.
18. Meyer RE, Liu G, Gilboa SM, Ethen MK, Aylsworth AS, Powell CM, et al. Survival of children with trisomy 13 and trisomy 18: a multi-state population-based study. Am J Med Genet A. 2016;170(4):825–37.
19. Nelson KE, Rosella LC, Mahant S, Guttmann A. Survival and surgical interventions for children with trisomy 13 and 18. JAMA. 2016;316(4):420–8.
20. Janvier A, Farlow B, Barrington KJ. Parental hopes, interventions, and survival of neonates with trisomy 13 and trisomy 18. Am J Med Genet C: Semin Med Genet. 2016;172(3):279–87.
21. Baty BJ, Jorde LB, Blackburn BL, Carey JC. Natural history of trisomy 18 and trisomy 13: II. Psychomotor development. Am J Med Genet. 1994;49(2):189–94.
22. Souka AP, Michalitsi VD, Skentou H, Euripioti H, Papadopoulos GK, Kassanos D, et al. Attitudes of pregnant women regarding termination of pregnancy for fetal abnormality. Prenat Diagn. 2010;30(10):977–80.
23. Chescheir NC, Cefalo RC. Prenatal diagnosis and caring. Womens Health Issues. 1992;2(3):123–32.
24. Rebagliato M, Cuttini M, Broggin L, Berbik I, de Vonderweid U, Hansen G, et al. Neonatal end-of-life decision making: physicians' attitudes and relationship with self-reported practices in 10 European countries. JAMA. 2000;284(19):2451–9.
25. Milstein J. A paradigm of integrative care: healing with curing throughout life, "being with" and "doing to". J Perinatol. 2005;25:563–8.
26. McGraw MP, Perlman JM. Attitudes of neonatologists toward delivery room management of confirmed trisomy 18: potential factors influencing a changing dynamic. Pediatrics. 2008;121(6):1106–10.
27. Stokes TA, Watson KL, Boss RD. Teaching antenatal counseling skills to neonatal providers. Semin Perinatol. 2014;38(1):47–51.
28. Kennell JH, Slyter H, Klaus MH. The mourning response of parents to the death of a newborn infant. N Engl J Med. 1970;283(7):344–9.

Chapter 31
Navigating Complex Medical Decision Making in the Pediatric ICU

Jaime Jump

Case Introduction

Dominic just celebrated his 11th birthday, making him the oldest living patient with both 22q11.2 deletion and CEDNIK syndrome [1], a neurocutaneous syndrome characterized by cerebral dysgenesis, neuropathy, ichthyosis, and keratoderma [2]. He meal preps with his mom on Sundays, plays wheelchair kickball at school, and tells stories with nonverbal communication.

Dominic is admitted to the quaternary academic medical center where he has been treated throughout his life. Over the past several months, he has been hospitalized multiple times for acute hypoxemic respiratory failure requiring endotracheal intubation and mechanical ventilation. Although he has been admitted to the PICU multiple times, this time is different, and he has been here now for over 1 month. He has failed extubation, and bronchoscopy reveals severe tracheobronchomalacia with airway collapse below a PEEP of 10. You are on the PICU team, and are worried about his prognosis and plan of care. His long-time pulmonologist shares these worries and she discusses with you and your team the need to perform a tracheostomy to keep Dominic alive.

Usual Approach

A family meeting is held a few days after Dominic's failed extubation and bronchoscopy. Dominic's parents, maternal grandfather, the ICU team, and his multiple subspecialists including the palliative care team and his long-term pulmonologist, Dr. M, are present. Dr. M runs the meeting due to her long-term relationship with

J. Jump (✉)
Department of Pediatrics-Sections of Critical Care and Palliative Care, Texas Children's Hospital, Houston, TX, USA

© Springer Nature Switzerland AG 2020   217
K. Aberger, D. Wang (eds.), *Palliative Skills for Frontline Clinicians*,
https://doi.org/10.1007/978-3-030-44414-3_31

Dominic's family. There is a palpable intensity in the room prior to the start of the meeting. Dominic's parents are noticeably worried and fidgeting under the table while Dominic's grandfather is teary-eyed.

The meeting begins with a long re-cap of Dominic's hospital course by Dr. M that includes Dominic's past medical history and a review of his new problems including results of his chest MRI and bronchoscopy. Dr. M then recommends a tracheostomy and mechanical ventilation. She also states that she feels this intervention would allow for Dominic to have a good quality of life outside of the hospital. The room is then silent.

The silence is broken by Dominic's mother, Anna, who asks multiple questions about the risks and benefits of a tracheostomy and other alternatives to this intervention for Dominic. She expresses concern about Dominic's quality of life after the tracheostomy, especially with his likely need for mechanical ventilation Dr. M rebuts that in her opinion, a tracheostomy is in line with their family's goals and that Dominic would otherwise have a premature death without this intervention. The risk and benefits of tracheostomy are glossed over and alternative pathways are not taken into consideration. The tracheostomy is performed, and the patient is placed into a long-term care facility.

Palliative Approach

A family meeting is planned to discuss Dominic's overall prognosis and plan of care. As the pediatric critical care attending, you plan the multidisciplinary meeting a few days ahead of time. This planned approach allows Dominic's parents to prepare questions and to invite other family members involved in decision making. It also allows you to review pertinent medical facts with Dominic's consultants and ask them to participate. On the day of the meeting, you plan a pre-meeting with all participants to discuss the logistics (Table 31.1).

Dr. M, although interested in running the meeting, expresses that she has been having a tough time processing Dominic's case and defers to you as the meeting facilitator. You discuss with your colleagues the two options for Dominic's plan of

Table 31.1 Organize a pre-meeting

This allows for time to discuss the logistics of the meeting, i.e., who will run the meeting and goals of the meeting. This avoids confusion, especially when the meeting is large. Consider SPIKES protocol [3] for communicating serious news

Step	Context
Setting	Prepare before the meeting
Perception	Assess how the patient/family views the medical situation
Invitation	Ask permission to talk about a sensitive topic
Knowledge	Provide the medical facts
Empathy	Attend to patient emotions
Strategy and summary	Determine a plan of action and discuss timing of next meeting

care moving forward. These options include placement of tracheostomy with expected long-term mechanical ventilation and long-term care placement, versus a compassionate extubation. Despite the agreeement to discuss these issues in the premeeting, many of your colleagues are uncomfortable during this discussion and avoid eye contact with your and the family [4].

Box 31.1 Objectivity Can Be Difficult When We Are Deeply Invested in Our Patients
Difficult encounters can elicit strong emotions in providers. This can be a challenge in the dynamic of any encounter. Providers should be encouraged to tend to their emotions and discuss their difficulty with these situations with their peers. The palliative care team can act as a good resource for providers in this situation [6].

There is a palpable intensity in the room prior to the start of the meeting. Dominic's parents are notably worried and fidgeting under the table. Dominic's grandfather teary is-eyed and appears to be holding back a flood of emotion.

Box 31.2 Expect Emotion and Empathize
Name emotion. Help Dominic's parents to process the emotion…"It must be so hard to deal with all of this…" [4] Understand nonverbal communication. Clarify interpretation of nonverbal cues. "I notice that you seem anxious, are you uncomfortable with what we are going to talk about today?" [7, 8]. Pause frequently and allow for silence during family meetings.

You begin the meeting with a short introduction around the room and acknowledge the palpable tension before you begin the meeting. "Thank you, Anna and Adam, for being here today. I can't imagine how hard this all is for both of you." Anna responds with, "Thank you Dr. Smith, we have been processing all of the events of Dominic's hospitalization and just want to make sure we make the right decisions for him that are in line with our goals for his quality of life." You ask, "What have you been thinking and talking about?"

Box 31.3 Seek First to Understand Before You Speak
Begin the family meeting with an open-ended question instead of repeating medical information. This allows you to assess both the factual and emotional understanding of the family of the patient's illness [5].

After some moments of silence, Anna and Adam share that they requested to meet with the palliative care team months earlier as they started to face the reality of Dominic's prognosis given his diagnosis and pattern of recurrent hospitalization. They also share that although Dominic does have a GJ tube, they have been very against adding too many technologies to Dominic's life. Rather than make an assumption about acceptability of quality of life, you ask what a good life for Dominic would look like to them. They stress the joy and importance of going to school, going for his afternoon walks, and swimming in the ocean in the summer. They are also able to verbalize that during recent hospitalizations they have felt pressured to pursue a tracheostomy but had many reservations. They talk about their strong Christian faith, of what comes after this life, and have valued chaplain visits as well as a close relationship with the palliative care social worker.

> **Box 31.4 Build a Bridge to Decisions**
> After first listening, then ask for permission to share medical information. Follow this up with a recommendation based on what you have learned about the patient/family's values, goals, concerns, and how interventions would fit into those contexts.

You give a brief summary of Dominic's concerning clinical situation and lay out the options you discussed in the pre-meeting. You state clearly that he will not survive without mechanical ventilation. You reassure the family that if their choice is to focus on comfort and allowing Dominic to have a natural and comfortable death, then you will do everything to make sure that he does not suffer. Your recommendation based on what you know of their goals and of the medical information is to pursue comfort measures. You then reassure them you will support them in whatever decision they choose to make for Dominic. You then allow time for questions.

Dominic's parents cannot reconcile Dominic's life on dependent on machines. His parents feel that he would suffer greatly if he were dependent on mechanical ventilation and had to live away from them in a long-term facility. They request more time to think, and in the meantime continue his current care in parallel with future considerations.

> **Box 31.5 Lean on Your Team**
> No single team member can provide for all of a family's needs by themselves. Chaplaincy, social work, child life therapy, music therapy, and various other roles all potentially meet different needs for a family. If the family already has a relationship with a particular team, enable continuity of care if possible. Likewise, learn from all team members' prior interactions with the patient/ family to gain insight into how better to care for the family.

Chaplaincy and the palliative team social worker continue to meet with Dominic's parents daily. After several days of more support and discussion, Dominic is extubated with the plan to support him with non-invasive positive pressure ventilation if needed for a time-limited trial. Dominic extubates successfully, utilizes NIPPV for a short period of time, and is subsequently weaned to room air. He is transferred to the floor. His parents meet with the local pediatric hospice agency, which, unlike adult hospice services, often allow for concurrent medical care, including intensive home-based treatments. Dominic returns home with hospice services in place.

Box 31.6 Pediatric Hospice Does Not Limit but Instead Expands Care
The Health Care Reform Act (HCRA-2010) includes a provision called Curative and Palliative Care for Children (CPCC) in Medicaid and CHOP. This provision, effective since 2013, allows children who are enrolled in these programs to receive palliative/hospice care in addition to curative treatment. Some hospice referrals in pediatrics will therefore allow for continuation of life-prolonging therapies (e.g., palliative chemotherapy, NPPV).

Dominic lives for 6 weeks at home until he develops an acute event that results in hypoxemic respiratory failure and dyspnea. During these weeks, Anna and Adam develop a close relationship with the hospice social worker and chaplain. These team members were able to guide them through several legacy and meaning-making activities. With acceptance and love, and grounded in their steadfast faith, Anna and Adam decide for Dominic to remain at home instead of returning to the hospital. His symptoms are aggressively palliated and he dies comfortably at home surrounded by his parents, loyal canine companion, and home nurses.

Takeaway Points
1. PREPARE! Adequate preparation of both the providers and the family for a family meeting can lead to more success in sharing information and eliciting goals of care.
2. UNDERSTAND BEFORE SPEAKING! Asking questions and responding to emotion opens up the conversation to the core issues, whereas prolonged medical updates and jargon do not.
3. ALLOW FOR SILENCE! Do not feel the need to fill the space with medical information. Silence allows a family time to process and wrestle with their emotions. Both need to happen before the conversation can move forward.
4. LEAN ON YOUR TEAM! Nobody can meet all of a patient/family's needs by themselves.

References

1. Hsu T, Coughlin CC, et al. CEDNIK. Phenotypic and molecular characterization of an additional patient and review of the literature. Child Neurol Open. 2017;4:1–6.
2. Cohen JL, Crowley TB, et al. 22q and two: 22q11.2 deletion syndrome and coexisting conditions. Am J Med Genet. 2018;176(10):2203–14.
3. Baile WF, Buckman R, Lenzi R, Glober G, Beale EA, Kudelka AP. SPIKES-A six-step protocol for delivering bad news: application to the patient with cancer. Oncologist. 2000;5(4):302–11.
4. VitalTalk. Addressing goals of care: "REMAP". http://www.vitaltalk.org/quick-guides. Accessed 21 Dec 2017.
5. Buckman R. Communication in palliative care: a practical guide. In: Doyle D, GWC H, MacDonald N, editors. *Oxford Textbook of Palliative Medicine*. 2nd ed. New York: Oxford University Press; 1998. p. 141–56.
6. Thurston A. A piece of my mind. The unreasonable patient. JAMA. 2016;315(7):657–8.
7. Quill TE. Recognizing and adjusting to barriers in doctor patient communication. Ann Intern Med 1989;111(1):51–57.
8. Hamilton C, Parker C. Communicating for results: a guide for business and the professions. 4th ed. Belmont: Wadsworth; 1993.

Index

The manufacturer's authorised representative in the EU is Springer
Nature Customer Service Centre GmbH, Europaplatz 3, 69115 Heidelberg,
Germany. If you have any concerns regarding our products, please
contact ProductSafety@springernature.com

Printed and bound by CPI Group (UK) Ltd, Croydon, CR0 4YY
29/04/2026
02099451-0008